MW00945464

HEALTHSPAN

A Functional Guide To
Living Long and Dying Young

DONGXUN ZHANG, BOB ZHANG
& DAVID KINCADE

To find out more about this book or the author, visit: www.intendedevolution.com.

ISBN-13: 978-1545322895
ISBN-10: 1545322899

Printed in the USA

TABLE OF CONTENTS

Foreword...vii

Introduction..ix

    Our Perceived Environment............................xi

    The Mind-Body Paradigm..............................xii

    Intended Evolution Fitness...........................xiv

Intended Evolution 1

    The Body as an Ecosystem 5

    Intentional Change 9

    Specialization and Flexibility........................11

    Physiology as Evolutionary Updates 15

    Intelligence as Flexibility..............................16

Healthspan as Health and Fitness 20

    Healing and Change in This Lifetime............20

    Healthspan Management................................24

    Emotion and Evolution..................................27

    Automatic or Semi-Automatic Responses.....29

    Lifespan..31

Modern Environmental Demands 33

    Stress as a Demand for Change......................34

    Mental Stress 36

    Lifestyle 40

Flexibility and Healthspan 44

Modern Problems 47

Fitness as an Environmental Demand 49

Jane's Fitness Today 51

Intended Evolution Fitness 56

Healthspan Strategies 61

Stable Environments 62

Long Lifespan as an Environmental Demand 65

The Constant Emergency Strategy 67

Sports and Long-Term Frameworks 70

Long-Distance Travelers: A Long Healthspan 72

Mind-Body Fitness And Medicine 75

Change and the Environment 76

Awareness and Information Sharing 78

Jane's Highly Evolved (Human) Intelligence 80

Planning 82

Virtual Environments 87

Updating Memory 93

Visualizations 95

Mind-Body Fitness and Medicine 96

The Intended Evolution Framework 99

Is There Optimal Functioning or Fitness? 102

Jane's IE Program 104

The Intended Evolution Health & Fitness Framework:

The Mind's "Scaffolding" 105

Jane's   Healthspan   Optimization   Framework

Visualization 106

Commentary 109

Why 150 or 160? 111

Weight Loss 112

    The Shake 113

    The Twist 116

    Twist & Shake Comments 117

Weight-Loss Theory 118

    Eyes 120

    Teeth 122

How Can We Best Optimize Our Virtual Environment

Capacity? 125

Summation 127

Conclusion 134

Who We Are 138

Endnotes 142

FOREWORD

Intended Evolution Fitness is a revolutionary new way of looking at health and fitness. It is meant to help the health and fitness community use a broad framework based on the body's internal intelligence when optimizing their current programs or creating new ones. We have also created a series of specific applications to fit within our framework and include some examples later in the book.

Originally invented more than ten years ago, intended evolution fitness (IE fitness) is based on the theory of intended evolution which, while already formulated at that time, was finally formalized in book form last year.[1] We've presented some of the theory as it generally relates to the fitness framework because we also believe it helps explain why the mind-body paradigm works and is so important in moving forward in health and fitness. We understand that some of the early information tends to be theoretical and somewhat dense—so we recommend that the reader feel free to jump directly to areas in the book applicable to their interests first and then use Chapter 1 as context for that information when needed.

A portion of the specific applications in the program that has been taught to date targets the endocrine system for use with metabolic disorders, including weight loss and diabetes.

Seeing related problems over and over in his clinic, this metabolism program was originally formulated by Dr. Dongxun Zhang for a patient who specifically asked what types of things she could be doing given her metabolism-related issues, including a genetic predisposition to diabetes.

While Intended Evolution Fitness has applications to target virtually every system in the body, the acute need for help in this area of healthcare has been building for decades, and this program brings groundbreaking ideas and unique, effective techniques to the health and fitness fields.

INTRODUCTION

Nothing in biology makes sense except in light of evolution.
—Theodosius Dobzhansky

Throughout human history, we have been confronted with—and have adapted to—many challenges in our environment. Each new age, or step, meant new challenges being faced and a variety of new strategies to deal with them. But there is a unique aspect to human evolution: the increase in speed with which the modern environment changes. Each age in human evolution brings faster and faster change. The current world is far removed from what humans encountered as little as one hundred years ago.

Never before has the environment we experience in our daily lives changed as quickly as the modern age.

As a result, our bodies did not necessarily evolve to optimally deal with the challenges that modern societies present to your average Jane and John. There are several factors related to this phenomenon that make modern challenges even greater than one might expect. For example, over time, mental activities have rapidly become more prominent than physical ones. Modern tools such as computers, appliances, and construction equipment have allowed us to specialize our activities—often toward less physical movement and effort in favor of more mental work.

At the same time, information available to us through communication and computer technologies has resulted in a vast increase in demand for planning, problem solving, decision making, and executing strategies. In a way, we could say that our day-to-day activities have shifted from what we can or need to do (based on traditional environmental challenges such as keeping warm or finding food) to what we could do or want to do, including making plans farther and farther into the future and making them more accurately. For example, with our basics taken care of as never before, we can plan for our future professions, or even those of our children.

Our Perceived Environment

When we say modern environments are changing faster than ever before, we mean not only what we normally think of as our environment—such as our physical surroundings—but we have to take into account *everything* we perceive. Furthermore, our perceptions themselves change over time as evolutionary changes gave us more choices about what we can do in any given environment. For example, even a single important physical change like the opposable thumb brought more ways to interact with our environment (not just push-pull or right and left, but also pinching, twirling, twisting, manipulating, etc.). Such a change resulted in new ways to experience, perceive, and understand certain things around us. For example, with the ability to grasp and manipulate objects, a rock or stick could become a weapon or tool.

We bring this up because, as far as the body and brain are concerned, new understandings of the environment amount to a *change* in the environment. Therefore, actual change in an environment *or* the changing perception of it results in "effective change" that a person must face. This is the case with any new knowledge that results in a change in the way things are perceived and shows why our modern world is "effectively" or relatively changing so rapidly. Each new technological change creates new paradigms and new understandings, and that means new adjustments have to be made to our lives.

In today's modern society, new "technological tools" have required modern humans to adapt to more change in a decade or two than what might have once taken thousands of years. Of course, we are also using modern tools and technology to alter the physical environment itself, which is also changing faster and faster.

These factors have resulted in a "snowball effect." As many people who work in technology know, because our environment evolves so quickly, we need to continue to look at it in a fresh light. New tools create change in our world, and that world affects us, including what we need to try to do and be.

Therefore, modern environments create a greater need than ever to understand the way the human body has evolved to adjust to change as it pertains to today's world. We should not fight the way our bodies evolved; they are what we have. Rather, we can work within our evolutionary blueprint and learn to adjust our ideas about health and fitness going forward. In this time of information overload, it is especially important that we take charge and manage our environmental input and not just passively allow today's rapidly changing environment to dictate how our bodies are affected as we go through life.

The Mind-Body Paradigm

A new health and fitness paradigm is emerging that looks at the internal workings of the body as intelligent cells and systems. How these systems perform, including their health, depends not only on our activities but also on our perceptions of—and mental response to—our quickly changing environment. The mind-body paradigm takes what modern biology is now uncovering and applies it to the human body: that every living thing, even single cells, are intelligent in their own ways and have memories.[2]

Chapter 1 discusses the body's internal intelligence according to "Intended Evolution" and how we can use it to our advantage. We'll explain why the mind-body paradigm works and is so important to the future of fitness, healthcare, and medicine. Although, of course, many modern changes to our environment—such as pollution or stress—have negative consequences that society needs to continue to reduce, we believe that it is possible in general to move forward by riding the wave of environmental change, not rejecting or fighting it. Current mind-body medicine and fitness is proving a valuable tool for not just fitness but healthcare as a whole and is being used in many prominent institutional settings.[3]

In this book, we will explore some of our modern health and fitness challenges and how they arose, and we will offer a broad and flexible framework that can be used for many aspects of health and fitness today. One goal is to take the mind-body paradigm to a new level, dramatically increase its potential uses, and offer some ideas for doing so.

For all the fantastic lifestyle advantages developed by our modern society, we also face the many new challenges to human health and fitness. While excellence in sports and fitness has long been important in most human societies, like everything else, they will evolve, and we believe it has never been more important than now that it merge with plans for our overall health.

Intended Evolution Fitness

We believe a general health and fitness framework should be based on the widest possible context—our entire lifespans and even our entire evolutionary history. We put forward these ideas in the hope that others can utilize them for their own health and fitness programs for individuals to take into their everyday lives. We have also included some limited examples based on programs we have developed for various systems—including the endocrine system—for weight loss.

In today's world, your average Jane or John spends much of the day at computers doing mental work with little physical movement, except perhaps to get lunch. This is simply a reality, and our evolutionary framework doesn't judge this or other modern activities as bad or good but rather as a new environment that differs from those in our evolutionary past.

For example, as a thirty-three-year-old manager at a software development company, Jane works long hours and also commutes thirty minutes each way to her company's offices. While she would love to "lose a few pounds," Jane thinks of herself as in pretty good shape. She forces herself to get to the gym to work out a few times a week and is also a regular at her weekly yoga class. However, over the past few years, she has found it more difficult to keep the pounds off and seems to need more and more coffee to get going in the morning.

Furthermore, like many people who try to be proactive about their health, Jane is bombarded with information about fitness, diet, and workouts to the point of being overwhelmed with new and improved versions of various workout techniques. We believe that there is often a disconnect between the actual goals someone like Jane has and the images of activities and lifestyles she sees in today's media.

We sometimes see a similar disconnect between what is commonly marketed as "fitness" and the actual health of the individual. Like Jane, many people really want to feel better and be "healthy," whereas "fitness" is often depicted as having a certain look or achieving certain statistics such as weight, body fat percentage, or the ability to achieve certain performance metrics like miles run or biked.

While we consider many such measurements and concepts to be useful benchmarks, we also think we have novel ideas that can take health and fitness much deeper than what is currently portrayed. We want Jane and her fitness professionals to explore formulating an individualized "evolutionary" framework for her in order to evaluate what she has been doing and can be doing now. Finally, we want to make some recommendations to help her achieve her goals. We view the many widely varying and detailed fitness and exercise programs as tools Jane can choose from, depending on what makes sense for her. In short, we want Jane to begin to manage her health and fitness for her long-term goals.

According to the theory of intended evolution, Jane's moment-to-moment choices and actions within her environment are major factors in the internal workings of her body, including how she feels and her overall health. Her surroundings are perceived consciously and unconsciously, evaluated based on her past memories—including who she is in her DNA—and her body adjusts accordingly. Jane can begin to understand how and why modern environments affect her health and take positive action. She can be proactive by training her intelligent inner systems to interact optimally with her environment rather than passively allowing her current stress-filled situations to dictate her health.

There is a well-known aphorism in the field of biology that says, "Nothing in biology makes sense except in light of evolution" (Theodosius Dobzhansky). We believe one needs to look at the big evolutionary picture to best understand human physiology, health, fitness, and mind-body medicine. Using this wide-scope approach, these activities are simply a slice of Jane's entire expected lifespan, which in turn is a slice of her evolution. While she began her life with the physicality and genes from her ancestors, they provided her with built-in flexibility to face changes in her current lifespan. Recent scientific findings have shown that this flexibility is greater than we previously thought. Topics such as tissue remodel, healing ability, and stem cell research all continue to point in this direction, even in areas once thought impossible, such as the heart and brain.[4]

The process of change in this lifetime is subjective (personalized); we each start with a different "who we are"—our evolutionary past. But within those limits, the key to managing life's changes is in "what we do": our choices and actions greatly affect what we become during our lives, including our health and fitness. When speaking of the framework of a long and healthy life, we believe that "fitness" should not be separated from health, and in fact, they are really one and the same. Further, health is not really discernible from lifespan, since ultimately, our health dictates how long we live.

Therefore, the Intended Evolution Fitness framework entails planning the entire "healthspan," meaning we want to keep functioning as optimally as possible for as long as possible. Everyone is different and has evolved with unique DNA, and we want Jane to utilize all the tools she has inherited to deal with today's environment in the most advantageous way for her health and healthspan.

Chapter 1

INTENDED EVOLUTION

The health and fitness concepts, forms, and visualizations we describe for Jane later in this book are based on a new outlook on how the human body (and life in general) works, as put forward in the book *Intended Evolution.*[5] While we don't go into all of the theoretical details here, we want to include some general concepts for the reader. Therefore, while this chapter is quite detailed and the relevance to health and fitness is contextual in nature, we believe the information is helpful in understanding the later material and recommend referring back as needed.

According to the concept of intended evolution, Jane's perceptions and intelligence are not really separate from her physical body; rather, they are intimately interconnected. For example, one of Jane's liver cells has its own intelligence with which it perceives its surrounding environment and acts accordingly, much like Jane does as she goes through life. Furthermore, each liver cell has relationships with neighboring cells in which information is shared, forming a team or group (e.g., "functional units" in physiology). In turn, each group forms larger groups, such as organs and systems—and finally, Jane, the whole person. Jane is actually the combination of intelligent, information-sharing relationships that evolved within their local environments and now make up the inside of her body.

Therefore, Jane is actually made up of many intelligent "little Janes," teams of little Janes, and teams of teams of little Janes. Finally, the largest team is Jane the whole person, and her sense of self is actually a combination of evolutionarily relevant information shared by her living, intelligent, internal systems. Furthermore, information that Jane perceives is translated inward and becomes part of the environmental information to which the internal body reacts.

Let's imagine the company Jane works for. As the head of her department—and perhaps a director—Jane's activities or communications are translated down to relevant departments and employees depending on their role or relationship within the company—how the company evolved, if you will. Relevant information also moves in the other direction, up the chain from individuals towards the directors.

One thing that immediately stands out when we speak of Jane the person is that, as far as Jane's awareness is concerned, most of what is going on internally is done automatically and goes unnoticed. What is often called *subconscious activity* is discussed later in this book; however, a basic description of the concept is that information moves in both directions with respect to the living relationships inside Jane's body and also moves subjectively based on her body's evolutionary past. We say "subjectively" because we aren't implying that Jane's liver cell has intellectual capacity like Jane; rather, it just reads local signals that come into its environment. However, these signals can originate from Jane's perceptions, like the fight-or-flight hormones that are produced and which signal action is needed when she perceives something frightening.

As another example, a sharp pain or discomfort may be translated directly to Jane's awareness, whereas information about a small internal change in blood pH or other homeostatic functions may only be relevant (and, therefore, perceived and adjusted) locally by the internal organs. What gets communicated—and where the communications go—is based on the evolution of Jane's internal systems. This kind of communication evolved in specific ways: internal systems are specialized to perform specific tasks, while energy, resources, and even the ability to process information are limiting factors. For example, the lungs need to know about demand for oxygen, the kidneys need to know about blood pH, and at the highest level,

Jane will generally only be made aware of internal happenings when her executive decision making is needed.

Using the previous "Manager Jane" example, her actions and communications vary and have subjective meaning to the various individuals or groups in her department depending on the relationships that have evolved within the company. One of Jane's actions might increase the workload and size of one department, cause another to rearrange itself or downsize, or not pertain to and therefore be ignored by yet another. Conversely, if an individual employee has problems, it becomes known through the channels that have developed (or evolved) over time. Perhaps this information reaches all the way up to Jane if it's important enough; however, most of the time problems are resolved at a "local level" without requiring Jane to become involved.

Certain practices in a company, like homeostasis in the body, can also become *automated* at local levels over time, even though they may have originated as management-level decisions years ago. As they are repeated over and over and are no longer regularly discussed at higher levels, these types of interactions are taken care of locally. They can also become harder to change over time as they become standard accepted practices. Such communication patterns are analogous to what we call "core" practices or systems when speaking of the human body; they've been re-enacted and "hardwired" for extended time periods with no need to change, even as the company (or body) changes at other levels. Again, this is advantageous because it allows the manager (Jane) to pay attention to other more important decisions, saving time and energy. Unless a big problem develops, it is inefficient to have a highly paid manager spending time on details that others are tasked with handling. All living systems are very efficient, and similar patterns of communication have evolved in the human body.

When we say that some internal systems "act automatically," we want to clarify that these are still intentional and intelligent activities at a given level of internal life. For example, during weightlifting, Jane's muscles "sense" the stress or demand on them and can send out signals to deliver more protein to increase their size if the demand persists over a long enough time period. But Jane isn't aware of all the local details; she simply perceives the internal signals relevant to her function as the manager, so to speak—such as a craving for her favorite protein dish, which she then seeks out. Therefore, we are not saying Jane is aware of—or using—her awareness and intending all these internal workings but only that they are being done intelligently at a given level. Basically, many internal activities have evolved to be taken care of immediately and locally with little to no input from time-consuming communication with Jane's awareness.

The Body as an Ecosystem

Although the inside of Jane's body may seem somewhat chaotic, complex, or "mechanical," it is important to realize that Jane's internal cells and systems are the result of intelligent activities and information sharing during her evolutionary past. Furthermore, they use that past evolutionary information (memory-DNA) to intelligently make decisions now. In other words, Jane's evolutionary past is the context for how her body reacts in this lifetime.

According to intended evolution, all organisms (including Jane) are made up of cooperative groups that share information and were selected during evolution as environments and situations changed. These evolutionary relationships, including their ability to adjust and change, underlie Jane's physical abilities and limitations as they pertain to her health and fitness. They also underlie her ability to change and repair problems that arise.

If you think about it, companies and other organizations like the one we use in the "Jane the Manager" example are also built on mutually beneficial relationships: employees get paid, and the company receives value from their work. While it may sometimes look like one group or individual is not benefiting from a certain viewpoint, there must be some benefit, or the relationship would be too unbalanced and break apart. Furthermore, like the human body, company relationships have some inherent "flexibility," or ability to be changed, depending on their nature.

Relationships or agreements create greater abilities (specializing for teamwork, for example) but also create limitations because they imply "rules" of engagement, so to speak. If the rules aren't followed, they have to be changed, or problems within the team—possibly even a breakup—might result. Like these relationships within an organization, it is the evolutionary history of our various internal relationships that dictates the range of their potential change going forward.

We could also say that evolution dictates the current "rules of physiology," which, therefore, demonstrates its importance to our health and fitness in this lifetime. For example, the heart has evolved for a certain range of function depending on the individual, and the flexibility within that range is also limited. We are all biologically complex individuals and can't just become anything we want. Certain body types and genetic traits may allow one to play professional basketball but not another, despite some inherent flexibility. Evolution has selected traits in us for not only the performance of a specific task but also the flexibility to adapt to new tasks and challenges that environment's present.

Early on in evolution (a few cells or colony of cells), maybe all cells would survive a breakup of their arrangement, since these simple relationships are very flexible and much less complex than higher organisms. But with complexity comes an increasing amount of reliance on one another, or what is called "specialization." Greater specialization means cells putting more resources into certain functions, which allows each to get better at what they do, benefiting all involved. Lung cells have become very efficient at collecting oxygen, which allows other organs to concentrate on their specialties; however, each now has limited functions. As complexity evolves, by definition, limitations are included in the specialization of cells in a relationship; any specialization means you rely on others so you can do so. Similarly, the people in Jane's marketing department couldn't focus strictly on marketing tasks if others didn't go out to sell the product and still others didn't produce it. Furthermore, those in the different departments have spent a lot of time to learn their specialty and may not have the flexibility to fill in at other jobs.

So, while our evolution has provided many amazing abilities and functions, it also includes some individual limitations. A good example of this is that some earlier lifeforms can build new or "regenerate" structures that are damaged or lost, but humans have lost the flexibility of these functions as more specialized attributes developed.[6]

Therefore, Jane's previous evolution dictates the mechanism and amounts of changes available to a given system during her lifetime. However, Jane *can* choose how to use her potential to change (what we also call flexibility) and try to enact change in a way that is as beneficial as possible.

According to *intended evolution*, Jane's evolution and current flexibility in her lifetime were influenced by experiences in her evolutionary past, and we want Jane to be able to take advantage of the benefits and not challenge limitations further than they evolved to be—or it may cause trouble. For Jane to achieve her maximum healthspan, it's good for her to understand some of the "rules" of the game, so to speak, that will help her reach her goals.

Intentional Change

According to intended evolution, if Jane's ancestors had to change their diet—perhaps because their environment changed and a new plant replaced a previously eaten one—their digestive systems would have attempted to change themselves to deal with the new food. Of course, behavioral decisions would also need to be made: use this plant, try others previously not eaten, or perhaps move to where the familiar plants still grow. Natural selection acts on these decisions: perhaps only some could tolerate the new plant and survive, or perhaps the ones who made the behavioral choice moved to a new area where it was still available.

But according to intended evolution, internal systems are intelligent, and if survival was possible, information about the new conditions was passed down for use in a future generation (see the book *Intended Evolution*). If these conditions persisted long enough (perhaps many generations), possible adjustments would be made to relevant systems—such as related digestive organs—and become permanent. Human jaws and teeth, for example, have been "downsized" over time with the decrease in need due to dietary changes, such as cooked food.

At Jane's company, when external forces demand that their product change, employees who make, sell, and market it may have to change their routines. If the new demand for change is not too dramatic, the company intentionally "evolves" over time (intended evolution), or if the company is highly specialized, it may end up not surviving (natural selection).

While this explanation of evolution by "intended evolution" (the passing down of acquired information from generation to generation, similar to J.B. Lamarck's ideas on evolution[7]) is not well accepted in science today, physiological change in this lifetime *is* well accepted, and that is important to health and fitness.

One example of intelligent internal change in this lifetime comes if Jane starts a weightlifting program to build muscle. Physiological changes can take time and repetition, so if Jane wants bigger muscles but only works out once, her body won't call for much protein to enlarge itself. But if time and repetition make it clear that a larger muscle is needed, change will begin. Her entire body is made up of intelligent systems interacting and changing based on their perceived environments (here, muscles sense added demand from the weights and send out signals for energy). Over time, her body could also reduce structures in certain areas that are not being utilized. This is what happens to muscles when someone is confined to a hospital bed for long periods of time or when astronauts spend extended periods in space.

Imagine Jane's department at work having a more compressed deadline than normal due to an important order. She gets the project done by making short-term adjustments, such as working overtime. Afterwards, the department pretty much returns to normal, unless such events keep repeating and she decides it makes sense to request an expansion of her department on a more permanent basis. The same applies to reducing her department; it isn't feasible to maintain its size if need decreases permanently, but Jane wouldn't reduce the department if the slowdown is thought to be temporary. Our internal systems also have memory and will change themselves based on evolutionary experience and current needs.

Finally, what we call core systems in Jane's body that haven't changed much and are more intertwined in newer systems or functions are harder to change than more flexible ones. Similarly, a company with a lot of history tends to have a lot of traditions and rules about how to do things, which are relatively inflexible because they have proven to work well over long periods of time.

Although cooperation and communication in the human body is much more complex than Jane's company—especially given its long evolutionary history—we believe similarities allow the analogy to give us useful insight into why and how to trigger the challenges needed to make the healthy changes Jane wants going forward.

Specialization and Flexibility

As previously mentioned, when two living things, such as cells, cooperate, this implies "specialization," whereby each individual puts more energy into one function and another need is met elsewhere, such as from others in the group. When information is shared, it allows all involved to specialize and improve at a particular task. Specialization is essentially the use of an individual's resources in a more focused way, allowing him or her to become better and more efficient at given functions. This occurs naturally if information is shared and is mutually beneficial to those involved.

However, this also results in some individual functions being reduced or eliminated in order to specialize in another, and this only occurs when those needs are met in some other way. For example, the brain needs to have nearly all its resource requirements met: energy by the digestive system, oxygen by the lungs, and delivery by the heart. This is not unlike upper-level decision makers at a company; they don't provide much actual input to produce the product; instead, they guide and make decisions. The human brain could not have evolved the way it did unless along the way its needs were met by other cells or systems.

Specialization of the workforce is a well-known concept in economics, as well. Each department in Jane's company is "specialized" and can do so because they have agreements, cooperate, and split up who performs which tasks. The marketing department can spend all its time honing its expertise on this one task because others make and sell the product, allowing them the benefit of pay without doing every task.

We can see how cooperation (information sharing) results in specialization and subsequently overall efficiency, but again, cooperation also reduces individual "flexibility" when compared to the state before the group formed.

When you get a job, you have certain hours and obligations and can't farm for your food anymore; in the body, brain cells also can't find their own food anymore. The extent of specialization and flexibility depends on the complexity of the system—the organ or the organism, for example. In humans, each organ pretty much needs the others to survive, whereas some lower lifeforms can regenerate various needed parts, a function we have lost in many cases. Therefore, while Jane's body has flexibility to make changes, this does not mean she can make any changes she wants; rather, she is limited by her evolution. That said, while our brain cells, being extremely specialized, may have little physical flexibility to change, some other cells and systems retain much more. Many cells in our bodies do have some flexibility for quite remarkable changes, including various types of stem cells, which are being found to be more plentiful than previously thought.[8]

We use the term "flexibility" often, by which we mean the general ability of biological systems to make changes to themselves as needed, including healing functions. The ability to adjust to change is built into all systems based on evolutionary needs and is also therefore limited based on that. Retaining unnecessary functions, including flexibility, is expensive in energy, resources, and potential that can be better used elsewhere, such as further specialization. This is not unlike Jane and her company: for her to keep practiced enough to be able to fill in for anyone in her department takes too much away from her management role. Therefore, others with similar roles maintain the ability to step in during their colleagues' absences, allowing Jane to specialize in management.

The need for Jane's body to change or adjust can come from any number of sources, such as physical damage, homeostatic rebalancing, attacks on the immune system, cell or system remodeling, or even exercise, all depending on the system involved. Each system, from an individual cell to organs and systems, all have limited flexibility in this lifetime, and we want to make sure Jane uses her flexibility wisely, since too much challenge can wear out any given system if demands are too great.

So, when we say Jane cannot just do or become anything she wants, this is because the flexibility of her internal systems is limited and saved in her DNA. Different systems of our bodies have different abilities to change (flexibilities) based on their evolutionary history, meaning their potential to repair and heal themselves is also limited. Furthermore, all systems and their functions ultimately interact or overlap; therefore, something causing one problem can affect our overall healing potential.

More on this facet of flexibility is discussed later, but basically, it is important to follow our evolutionary "blueprint" (DNA) if we are to maximize our health. This can be considered the baseline we work off of as individuals, which also gives us some of our individual attributes and talents.

Physiology as Evolutionary Updates

During the course of human evolution, newer functions and relationships often arose as updates to current systems were needed. New needs were often met by the current cells or systems changing their size or functions or taking on a support role for a newer system. The human brain has many examples of newer functions and structures being "layered over" old ones, so to speak, or by co-opting structures for new functions.[9] The vascular structures (like the heart) that supplied the internal systems with resources earlier in our evolutionary past have changed themselves over time as needed.

Notice we are not saying that internal cells or systems know about the whole body; in fact, the opposite is true. Local systems adjust to local demands and work within immediate larger constraints, including time and energy availability. This is what we mean when we say Jane can't just become whatever she might imagine: her body can't start over (like constructing a new office building exactly how she imagines), but rather, the intelligent internal systems start with what they have and update when possible based on what is demanded of them. This can be seen as analogous to Jane's office building: when they need to expand her department, they can't just add a new floor or even make the current floor bigger; they have to work with the current core structure to some extent.

That said, some of this type of flexibility is also present in Jane's current lifetime: vessels of the heart will attempt

15

to grow around a blockage, for example.[10] Healing examples like this are responses to environmental demands—or, we could say local conditions—and occur all the time in the body. Of course, flexibility in this lifetime is limited compared to changes during evolution. However, the body still possesses remarkable capabilities in healing injuries and illnesses, even later in life. Flexibility in this lifetime is directed towards what Jane has now, healing and adjusting what she has in this generation and not trying to make too many major changes like we see during evolutionary time periods.

Intelligence as Flexibility

Whereas many animals have physical "specialties" to find food and avoid trouble (speed, claws, flight), humans evolved dexterity (hands) followed by intelligence as our main specialty in dealing with the environment. "Core" systems (like homeostasis) take a supporting role to allow intelligence to work optimally with respect to external demands without having to pay too much internal attention. Therefore, as Jane moves through life and challenges arise, she is meant to deal with them by the newest and best source of flexibility—primarily, her modern human intelligence.

The reader will note that we are listing the brain (a very specialized organ) as a source of flexibility, although it is not known for the ability to repair itself like some organs or tissues—rather, the opposite is true. Furthermore, we said above that flexibility is the ability of a system to change itself based on environmental demands. While the brain, including the details of memory and processing, is complex and best left to those who study it, we believe information must make internal changes in some way to create or change our memories, and therefore, the brain actually provides an amazing flexibility with respect to our interactions with our environment. For example, compared to any other system, it specializes in rapid processing of information and updating of memory, all in huge volume, giving humans the ability to quickly understand new situations and formulate new plans to avoid or adapt to environmental change. Therefore, we look at the modern human brain, perhaps evolution's newest and most specialized invention, as adding the most flex potential to the human as a whole.

Interestingly, our advanced mental capacity allows us to avoid as much physical challenge as possible. While the regenerative capacity of simpler lifeforms seems almost miraculous in some ways, such as when we see the ability to regrow tails, claws, or even limbs, our modern brain and human circulatory system might not have been possible if those functions were retained. When functions and structures were updated over and over in order to specialize towards intelligence, some physical flexibility was lost, and some systems became more fixed. But intelligence allowed the ability to avoid many challenges and regeneration, and other physical alterations were no longer of much advantage compared to the increase in intelligence. This is important to Jane's fitness because it is her intelligence that is meant to be her primary tool in dealing with her environment, and her available physical flexibility should be applied wisely and intentionally.

What we are saying here is that human intelligence allowed avoiding many physical challenges and replaced much of the need for physical change. Essentially, Jane's physical flexibility is limited because her intelligence became the function to deal with challenges from the environment. Interestingly, it is also intelligence that allows her to have some control over her how she uses the flexibility she does have and, as the reader will see, is the basis of the intended evolution fitness framework.

We could say that every person has a sort of "fitness possibility tree" of varying size and makeup, depending on his or her individual constitution (evolutionary history in the DNA). The support structures (trunk and large branches) aren't very flexible and shouldn't or can't be forced to change much, but newer, more flexible growth (leaves and flowers) can make big changes. All people and each of their internal systems have their own unique *flexibility-stability ratio*, and so managing the various systems of the body is key to the maximization of health.

Jane's highly specialized intelligence functions not only allow her to avoid trouble today but also to plan far into the future for what is coming. We often take this function for granted, but it is of tremendous benefit for herself and, of course, for her internal systems.

This ability to plan is the basis of the intended evolution fitness framework. It allows her to intentionally and purposefully plan for a long, functional current lifespan in the direction of her choice. She can create a plan, or *blueprint* for this lifetime, to optimally match her initial DNA blueprint. When she plans a long, healthy lifespan (we say long "healthspan"), her intelligent internal systems will also begin to use their flexibility potential to adjust and do their part to make it happen.

Chapter 2

HEALTHSPAN AS HEALTH AND FITNESS

As she moves through her life, we want Jane to take into account that each body starts with a limited ability to change and heal itself over time. In order to effectively manage this limited flexibility potential, it is important for her to take into consideration her short- and long-term goals, as well as her overall lifestyle.

Healing and Change in This Lifetime

One result of the updating through evolution is that the body's most recent changes tend to be the most flexible and adaptive with respect to the outside world, whereas those that have been stable and less challenged throughout evolution tend to be what we call "core" systems or functions. Core systems became the "backbone" of the newer ones and include homeostatic systems such as the internal organs, which provide support to keep the environment stable for the systems that interface with the outside world. So, evolution of internal life is about moving forward with what it had at the beginning, not just based on a theoretically "best" structure.

Our examples are generalizations, but they give us clues about how change occurs in our bodies when they are challenged, including the fact that when that change occurs, it is meant to happen "from the outside in," so to speak. The most flexibility is found where environmental demands historically changed, such as in systems that continue to interface with the ever-changing external environment (skin, limbs, muscles, intelligence). What we call deeper or "core" systems tend to have stable interior environments, have other functions "layered" on top of them, and are less flexible to change (internal organs). Of course, all systems have some flexibility, such as healing potential, and the term "core" is relative. For example, we know each organ has its own unique ability to repair in limited ways. We simply find the term "core" useful to speak generally about these concepts.

Therefore, we look at the activities Jane chooses—including her specific fitness programs—as planned slices of her entire lifespan, which, in turn, is a slice of her evolution. She needs her specific fitness activities to fit within a context, or framework, for her overall health goals to be most effective. Furthermore, when we talk about and plan Jane's health and fitness goals, we want to focus not just on maximizing her lifespan but maximizing what we call her "healthspan"—maintaining her *needed functions* in good working order for as long as possible, given who she is along with her goals going forward. During her evolution, important structural and functional information was saved (DNA), including information about her lifespan as a whole and that of each individual unit.

This does *not* mean that one's lifespan or healthspan is fixed; as we said earlier, there is flexibility built into our systems. However, saved lifespan information and its interface with the current environment are both very important to the formation of realistic expectations needed to plan optimal functionality and maximum healthspan.

As we have said, the ability for Jane's body to change and adapt—what we have been calling her "flexibility"—is limited; she can't make unlimited demands on her body to change. This makes intuitive sense because we know she can't live forever. Limited lifetimes also follow from our assertion that our limited ability to heal is part of the flexibility or adaptability factor. Healing is essentially the ability of a given system to change or repair its condition and, therefore, part of Jane's evolved flexibility and lifespan equation. Used-up flexibility (potential to change) eventually leads to lack of function and, when severe enough, the end of that function. This is an important issue when speaking of Jane's potential quality of life over time.

An important feature of the body's flexibility potential, and a main theme of this book, is that core systems, such as the kidneys, have less ability to repair and change than the systems which are meant to interface with changing external environments. This is directly related to their specialization and role in functions such as homeostasis, which are meant to be protected by using our intelligence. Therefore, we don't want Jane to continually challenge any system beyond its natural capability to perform, and this is especially important with core systems. Furthermore, core systems are also dependent on each other, so it only takes one to be compromised or fail for serious problems or even death to occur.

In the broad picture, the only thing life—including our internal systems—can't overcome is continuous change, and since change is endless, the changing environment that shapes life also eventually ends it. But Jane can—to some extent—control her response to environmental demands for change and therefore affect her health, fitness, and healthspan. We want Jane to plan for, or manage, these continuous changes by anticipating and planning for what will come and to direct her body's potential going forward. We call this *cumulative directional progress*, meaning she can use her flexibility, or potential for change, to move her towards her goals—including the goal of a long healthspan and avoiding unneeded use of her flexibility potential when possible.

Healthspan Management

An important factor that affects Jane's healthspan is her choices and actions in dealing with her ever-changing environment: how she manages her life. All organisms, including Jane, use their flexibility to deal with life's challenges, but Jane and other humans can choose, or manage, how they do so. Therefore, careful planning or managing of her responses to life's challenges, or environment, can be highly advantageous going forward.

For example, in a well-run company, throwing money at every project makes little sense. As Jane moves through life, making choices as she goes, these choices slowly determine what her constitution (genetic makeup or DNA) did not: what Jane does *every moment* in her life also affects her internal makeup and her future. Over time, Jane's internal systems monitor their (internal) environments, just like she does the external environment, and use the information to make choices. For example, during her development, Jane's internal cells and systems turned off previous possibilities in their DNA[11] to focus on what was relevant: the internal environment being experienced in this lifetime. While this was most prevalent during development when Jane was very young, it continues to some extent throughout her life, and it is part of what we call her "loss of flexibility" as she ages. Unused functions tend to be downsized from lack of use, properly used functions tend to remain viable, and overused functions tend to wear out. Basically, the intelligent systems in the body will perceive a lack of demand for given functions and scale back their activity and potential, whereas overused ones can no longer make the necessary changes needed to return to baseline and will change their level of functioning or even form (e.g., scar tissue).

Even with normal functioning, over time, limitations can become greater and greater and flexibility less and less as abilities are dropped or reduced. This is a natural part of development and also of the aging process, but Jane's activities are important factors in how this process plays out for her healthspan going forward.

We want to emphasize that this is not necessarily a negative process; as we grow and specialize in life, it would be a waste of energy to keep all previous potential for all possible functions. Again, we see this most obviously during development, where previous flexibility is turned off as needs for it diminish. The body directs resources and flexibility where they are needed—where Jane focuses her attention, energy, and activities. This process is not unlike the "specialization" process we noted when speaking of development and evolution. Our bodies and mental capabilities also continue to specialize throughout our lifetimes. As we've said, we don't believe Jane's body is separate from her perceptions, intelligence, and intentions, so internal changes happen based on what she does *as well as* on what she intends to do in the future. Furthermore, we believe Jane's mental abilities, including memory, are her major source of flexibility in dealing with her environment as she moves through life.

For example, humans, including Jane, are born without knowing a language or having a profession, although there may be predispositions for talents in these areas. Jane grew up in the United States speaking English, went to school specifically for business, and then, over time, moved into a management position. These are all possible due to her mental flexibility in this lifetime, a unique human trait, but at the same time is an example of using mental flexibility to make choices to specialize. Conversely, we could also say these are examples of creating limitations as she moves through life.

Each advancement or specialization during her life meant giving up other options (decreasing flexibility). We are not saying these specializations are negative; managed planning in a given direction clearly allowed her to excel in school and benefited her in life, including in regards to her long-term goals. But what we start with (our DNA) and the choices we make about our activities over time *do* limit what we can do going forward.

Jane's DNA enabled her to choose between several sports at a high level in college, and she chose basketball. An example of flexibility and limitations is that she may have been able to choose another sport and excel to high levels if she had started young enough, but at some point, her end goal of playing at a nationally-ranked school meant choosing only one sport in her case.

Limitations are also based on end goals. If Jane simply liked athletics and viewed them as just a fun activity, she probably could have played several sports at a lower level and gotten quite proficient at each. We bring this up because our lives work in a similar way: flexibility and limitations are built based on evolution and this life's experience.

Using the analogy of Jane's company: perhaps it could transition from one type of software design to another—maybe—but it couldn't necessarily become an auto manufacturer without an unusual amount of time and resources. Life works this way, too. You can shift, but you have "expression limits" that increase as we move through life. For many people, use of their flexibility to make a lot of changes may not be optimal if they are looking forward to a long healthspan, especially if the changes will need to be reversed later.

Emotion and Evolution

Emotional states, including stressful feelings, involve communication pathways that have developed during evolution by repeated use of advantageous behaviors—to ensure escape to safety, for example. Therefore, while unhealthy when Jane experiences them too often or over extended periods of time, the origin of emotional and stressful feelings are a natural call for change or adjustment given a certain situation. When threatened, it was advantageous to have a very fast and strong anger or fear response for survival purposes, which return to baseline quickly after the danger is past. But these responses are not meant to be used too often or for long periods of time, which can create health problems. We will speak further on the unconscious or automatic aspect of these responses as well as habits, reflexes, and instincts in the next section and stress-related health problems in the next chapter.

At Jane's company, there might be a spike in demand for a product, creating a situation where everyone tries to help out by working long hours or even doing different jobs until the situation is rectified. If things return to normal in a reasonable time, it doesn't create long-term problems, and there is little need for permanent change. But if this environment persists and people are continually asked to change their routines—or even change them too quickly—problems will arise as people get angry. If there is no return to baseline, permanent changes may result as people quit or demand higher pay.

Demands that push functions to their normal limits, including emotions, keep us strong, healthy, and ready for performance. Furthermore, using functions in this way allows them to learn and get better (more efficient). However, wear, tear, imbalances, or pathologies result from pushing too often or too far, and not pushing enough or often enough is also a call for change and can create problems (for example, atrophy).

While a simple example of physically pushing too far would be joint wear and tear, this relates to many problems, from dietary to mental and emotional situations. Jane's mental capabilities are also rooted in the rest of her intelligent body, such as producing communication hormones that change when challenged and then (hopefully) revert to their healthy baseline.

Not only do we each have our own natural flexibility levels for dealing with change (both physical and mental), but so do our various internal systems based on their evolution. Each functional system will have its own stress points—limits of healthy use versus too much or too little—and any given activity will challenge different systems to differing degrees. For example, of major concern today is the overuse of the stress response compared to its evolved capabilities.

Other examples of environmental challenges that could be too far outside our ability to change are such things like pollution, toxins, or unrecognized dietary factors. Essentially, we believe such things can confuse the affected systems (and hence, also affect mental function) because they weren't environmental factors recognized and processed during evolution.

Automatic or Semi-Automatic Responses

According to Intended Evolution, our (somewhat) automated functions, including reflexes, instincts, emotions, and habits, were and are developed based on repeated reactions to choices. During evolution, for example, repeated activity such as running from a predator—or even the running activity itself—became more automated, or "hardwired," over time. We use the word "automated" in the sense that these decisions to act are made by various systems locally (for example, a reflex doesn't need to be thought about consciously) and, through repetition, became very efficient and fast through evolutionary time periods. Presumably, this is simply because actions repeated over and over don't need processing by the person's awareness since that processing resulted in the same decision each time. We can also see that the same thing happens in our current lifetime: when something is repeated over and over, we begin to do it automatically with little if any thought involved.

Therefore, efficiencies like reflexes, instincts, or habits arose naturally through repetition. Once established, these tend to lock a system into a process that has been experienced so often, or is so important, that the reaction develops to be done automatically. Like any increase in efficiency, it becomes a limiting process, which can be difficult or impossible to change depending on the history of the process. For example, we could say a given muscle reflex has a long evolutionary history and may be impossible to change, whereas a habit Jane acquired growing up (depending on the nature of it) may be more easily changed.

Emotions are another example of relatively automated responses where external stimuli and information are translated inward for the body to take action, followed by the appropriate movement of information back into the awareness. Perception of something dangerous, for example, will bring an internal release of fight-or-flight signals by relevant systems creating the potential for very quick and powerful action without much processing at the "person level." For many people, food can be similar—certain smells or visual cues can signal the digestive system to begin working to be ready for food.

Within our framework, these things aren't looked at in a negative way, but rather as evolutionary time-saving devices to allow our awareness and intellectual power to pay attention to new and more important information and not be bothered by repetitive activities. So, what Jane calls "bad habits" actually made sense to her body at the time they were formed, since they are a repetition of behavior that required fewer and fewer decisions and were taken over by local systems to continue into the future.

Lifespan

We put forward earlier that we view Jane's time doing fitness programs as slices of her lifespan and her lifespan as a slice of her evolutionary journey. According to the theory of intended evolution, a main activity of living things is collecting information and making internal adjustments, or updates, to best fit their expected environments going forward.[12]

For example, to simply survive, Jane's ancestors went through many changes. Their systems also made changes to themselves, or evolved, based on what was demanded of them. This is why one environment may be beneficial to one organism or person but not for another. Jane's internal systems may have evolved to meet challenges somewhat differently than some of her coworkers.

For example, people have widely varying food preferences and tolerances because of the information about their differing diets saved in their DNA. Dietary change also fits into our framework; taking the healthspan view, it points to different diets for different people so as not to push related functions past their "flexibility cap," so to speak.

Therefore, Jane's fitness and healthspan has a lot to do with new challenges and not demanding too much change in any function, including reduced use, which can cause atrophy, also a change and use of flexibility potential. What Jane perceives and what she does in her current environment—this lifetime—is very important to her health and fitness. Similar to the way Jane's company's overall success is based on current success as well as estimates about new and changing conditions going forward, Jane's healthspan will also be based on current conditions *and* her intentions and plans for the future.

Chapter 3

MODERN ENVIRONMENTAL DEMANDS

Jane's body has many intertwined functions, and when we say "demand too much change," this can mean many things depending on which function or system is being challenged and how. In this chapter, we will discuss some of the more flexible functions Jane wants to use to meet environmental demands along with the relatively inflexible core functions she wants to protect and not stress.

In today's world, humans control many factors of the environment that used to regularly challenge us. For example, modern living conditions like using houses for shelter, traveling in cars, working at desks, and eating processed foods have all changed the demands on Jane's body when compared to even her recent ancestors. Furthermore, sedentary lifestyles and information overload are assumed to be "the new normal," but with evolution as our guide, we don't believe these things are necessarily ideal given what she evolved to deal with.

The human body will try to change to keep up with its changing environment as best it can, but if excessive change is attempted, this may not lead to an optimal healthspan. As we shall see, there are things Jane can do to better match her body's evolutionary needs to the rapidly changing environment of today.

Stress as a Demand for Change

Theoretically, one could view stress as anything that challenges the body to change. Looked at in this way, not all stress should be viewed in a negative light. For example, "stressing" muscles can result in them becoming larger, which may be needed to meet demand. In our view, what is commonly viewed as stress (in the mental pathological sense) are demands that overload Jane's mental systems and aren't really resolved but instead build tension. Here, there is a call to action without progress towards a choice of action—no finality. More generally, we could say that most stress results from challenges that demand more change than one can handle in a timely manner.

These challenges or stresses can be found at various levels in the body. Jane may not always be aware that something she ate is challenging her digestive system, for example, unless it reaches a threshold where she notices some pain or discomfort. If her digestive cells are stressed, they do the best they can to use their flexibility to make adjustments in order to deal with the situation.

We will address physical stresses later, but we want to point out that this still involves intelligent activity happening at various local levels that can be relayed to our awareness, if strong enough. One may notice many discomforts due to local "physical" stresses in various parts of the body. The term "listen to your body" fits well in our framework because the mind arises out of—and is not separate from—the body, and therefore, naturally local trouble can be part of our awareness if severe enough.

Although we are not experts on the professionally accepted definitions, we think of mental stress (in the pathological sense) as *not* returning to balance, or baseline, in a normal time frame after, for instance, an emotional event. This entails any number of physiological factors not returning to baseline in a timely (normal) fashion.

When any part of Jane is unable to change or doesn't have the flexibility to meet new or even existing environmental demands, pathologies can begin to develop. This tends to especially accelerate if demands constantly keep the overall system out of balance—for example, chronic mental stress. When Jane says she is "stressed out" (lasting portions of a day or perhaps even longer), she is experiencing a situation that keeps the body out of balance for a time period and, to a degree, not planned for over her evolutionary history. In other words, there is no resolution to the calls to action because there is too much information that falls outside her ability to process. When this persists and headway isn't being made, feedback is unclear, gets muddled, and creates confusion in her systems.

Over time, unwanted changes can occur as a given cell or system does its best to adjust itself to these new yet persistent signals. These changes, while making sense at that local level because of the local conditions, may also be what we call a pathology when looked at from our viewpoint. For example, a smoker's lung cells can change from one cell type (ciliated type, which sweep mucus away, for example) to other types in response to the change to their environment (becoming a smoker).[13] While a problem for the person and their lungs going forward, the new form makes sense to the local cells given the constant smoke they have to deal with.

Mental Stress

As we have said, one cause of Jane's mental stress is essentially a backup of unprocessed or unresolved information (e.g., problems), which she continues to process so action can be taken. This so-called "stressed-out" state, or "information overload," is not surprising given the large increase in brainwork experienced today compared to even one hundred years ago. This is an important example of Jane's current environmental information not matching her evolution, and it's a major cause of health problems today. Interestingly, this is also a target of many mind-body programs, both historically (yoga) as well as in institutions around the country.[14]

Although the idea that perceptions affect physical health has long been assumed in Eastern cultures,[15] in the modern scientific paradigm, the study of the effects of stress has been a main link to this idea becoming more generally accepted. Although it is difficult to scientifically link a stressful situation to a given disease, it has become clear that stress can be a contributing factor to many disease states.[16]

Using the intended evolution framework—the idea that mental aspects and the body aren't really separate—this makes perfect sense: stress is subjective to the person experiencing it based on his or her internal makeup—and, therefore, perception. Jane may react quite differently to a given stressor than one of her coworkers due to the different evolution of their internal makeup: the perceptions and reactions of her internal systems. The same event that makes her angry might make another worried or fearful, while yet another may not be stressed at all.

The general takeaway as to the importance to health and fitness is that our perceptions of the outside affect hormones produced in the brain and elsewhere,[17] potentially affecting the entire body depending on the situation. Our perceptions therefore affect the entire endocrine system, which affect everything from emotions, sex, stress response, and even eating and drinking. Furthermore, as we have stated earlier, communication moves in both directions: for example, we know that hormones involved in changing internal states, such as those involved in emotions, affect our perceptions.[18]

Therefore, when formulating one's individualized framework, it also makes sense that everyone may choose different aspects of health and fitness. Knowing that Jane's perception is the interface of environmental information with her internal systems also makes sense of the idea of stress as an evolutionary tool (developed because it was helpful) used by her body for her benefit (e.g., fight-or-flight). Emotions and stress can be called an evolutionarily important and natural call to action by the body to our awareness that something is happening needing immediate action, so the fact that these reactions often require little thought was advantageous during evolution.

Jane and her coworkers are experiencing an environment that includes a large increase in calls to action compared to their evolutionary past, even those as recent as what their grandparents experienced. Therefore, a dramatic increase in stress-related health problems is not surprising.

Jane's emotional responses occur as a result of what she perceives to be important information, which needs quick action. Once processed, she should return to a balanced state, but often in her job, she is subjected to a high volume of such information. If too much time is spent re-acting rather than at baseline, it can create undue demand for change (here in body chemistry) and too much use of her flexibility or change potential in those systems. In to-day's world, emotional and stressful responses to environ-mental stimuli are increasing rapidly, and stress is becom-ing one of the most talked about problems in healthcare.

It is interesting to think that humans, who have evolved to be wary of and have emotional responses to things like wild animals or other physical threats, respond to workplace problems with similar responses, even though no real physical threat exists. This is a wide-ranging topic, and we are not experts in psychology, but we pre-sume that any alarming or threatening information can cause such a response, including things learned in this life-time.

While this may seem a bit deterministic, as if there is nothing Jane can do but grin and bear her emotional stress, she can use the knowledge that her systems and their mem-ories are, and can still be, updated in this lifetime to her advantage. Just as memory is updated with environmental change, Jane can update hers proactively, as we will discuss shortly.

A common example of this with respect to stress is that a doctor may recommend some time off, which essentially brings new information in and allows unresolved infor-mation or problems to be processed. In the next section, we will discuss the human mental ability to plan, visualize, and create what we all a "virtual environment" as a way to update our memory systems to actualize a plan that can be used to avoid stress if used properly.

Given Jane's current goals, the use of long hours of brain work on her computer may be her best way to achieve maximum earnings power. In other words, "working hard" maximizes her profit. But she has to be careful to also balance her activities to keep her important functions in a range that optimizes her health and healthspan.

For example, Jane's company could be putting effort into sales to keep money flowing in, but too much focus on sales could create a backlog while trying to process the orders. Employees from other departments could get stressed and angry and start to complain about all the resources going to sales. Like Jane, the company wants a long future ahead of it and doesn't always want to sacrifice the long-term for short-term gain, except in special circumstances.

Similarly, Jane has to take care of the relationships with her living internal support ecosystem, or stress will develop, endangering her long-term health. Constant demand on emotional responses, such as fight-or-flight, is no different; eventually, related glands and organs will wear out, just like a knee or shoulder joint.

Lifestyle

Too little use of some systems, such as those involved with movement (a sedentary lifestyle), is also a major problem in today's world. We could look at this as a lack of challenge or environmental demand compared to what we evolved for. Evolution provided for a certain range of activity, both mental and physical. In today's modern societies, there is little need to utilize some of our evolutionary functions for everyday living. This is part of the problem with Jane's current environment: lack of demand for some of her movement functions and too much demand for her mental functions, both of which we will address in formulating her program.

If we look at Jane's body as an ecosystem, or even a company with various departments, we consider a sedentary lifestyle to be an environmental challenge on some of her systems. This is because it also results in demand for change when compared to what is evolutionarily within the normal functioning limits of some of her systems or "departments." Lack of activity and a high caloric intake both send signals to the body that related evolutionary functions need to be changed.

For example, decreased demand for movement functions means those functions can be downsized while increased digestive and storage capacity (fat) functions need to be increased. We feel both of these are examples of functional needs currently being stretched beyond normal evolutionary flexibility capacity and will shorten lifespans in the future. Challenges to functions such as these, and the body's resulting attempts to make needed changes, can be at the expense of future capacity to change and repair.

Again, looking at Jane's company as an analogy, if their business environment changes, of course they need to make changes to reflect that. If the employee agreements are out of balance within the company and some feel the situation is no longer mutually beneficial, they can alter their behavior, demand change, or leave. Perhaps adjustments can be made, but the capacity for change is not unlimited, so good management and wise choices need to be made for the future of the business if it is to continue to function.

One might ask why Jane's internal storage systems would pack on fat and gain weight if it is unhealthy for her as a whole? Why is it mutually beneficial for fat tissue to take up so much of the body's resources and flexibility potential for the many people suffering from the obesity and diabetes epidemic we see today? Of course it isn't, and that's the problem: the pathologies associated with weight gain today are an example of internal systems becoming out of balance and attempting to change and rearrange their function levels and structure and, in some cases, wearing out from overuse. The flexibility potential for some functions allowed in the DNA blueprint are stretched beyond capacity, and the related systems are trying to change the normal behavior for which they evolved.

Jane evolved this way because lack of activity, a sedentary lifestyle, or high mental stress is all a relatively new experience, or environmental condition, and doesn't match Jane's evolution. For humans, dietary challenges in past environments had to do with not having enough food rather than too much, and that was the main challenge in life.

Therefore, not only was internal flexibility directed to finding and storing scarce resources, but instinctual behaviors also developed to make this very important process more efficient. Historically, too much food and gaining too much weight was not a big problem for the vast majority of people.

We might even say that people who have a hard time dieting today may very well have been quite evolutionarily fit in this respect, and they may be here today because of this instinctual behavior in the past! Basically, Jane's ancestors had to become very good at gathering and storing (fat) resources in order to carry an energy source with them to take advantage of good seasons or bountiful times. The ability to store fat and become overweight or obese in today's world is actually a reflection of how important resource storage was evolutionarily and can also be reflected in genetic differences.[19]

Modern overconsumption causes the digestion and energy storage systems to become stressed by overuse, resulting in the inability to cope normally, and leads to metabolic disorders such as diabetes and obesity. Even if she can burn it off during her younger years, as Jane's body changes and her metabolism slows, her earlier habits can become a problem later in life. It is therefore important for Jane to be the manager of her life, plan ahead for what she wants going forward, and match her current short-term activities to fit her long-term goals. She needs to be aware that her evolutionary past and the instinct to eat was made for a different age but is still in effect today. We often see that willpower or motivation to burn calories or stop eating is a prominent theme in today's popular media, but as we will see, changing one's environment and retraining the body can be a powerful addition to that strategy.

Flexibility and Healthspan

Intelligent internal systems are a bit like communicating teams in that they can get stressed by each other's abnormal or inconsistent activity. Trouble with one system (e.g., an organ) can affect many others, and if this stress persists, it can begin to alter behavior. So, while we can view extra fat as just that, what is often called a "metabolism imbalance" or disorder is an example of how changing or imbalanced internal relationships can affect other systems at some point. For example, processing and storing an overabundance of calories leads to fat building up in organs and the vascular system, creating unhealthy environments in all those affected areas. Even Jane's intelligence, being rooted in these systems, is not exempt, and such trouble can also affect mental performance (lethargy, lack of concentration, hormone imbalance, etc.).[20]

A straightforward and common example of pushing a function beyond its ability to change and repair normally (flexibility) is the overuse of a knee joint, resulting in an altered structure, impairment, or even a replacement being needed. Of course, interventions such as joint replacements are proven tools for given problems and extend good functionality, but we do view the conditions that led to their need as a reduction in healthspan. Naturally, we would all like to avoid such intervention if possible because overall, there is loss of optimal function going forward.

Compared to limbs, though, the problem with stressing a more *core* structure or function, such as an organ, is that organ relationships are more tightly interrelated (homeostasis, for example) and rely on each other more fully than do peripheral ones. You can't lose too much function in any organ without the rest also being affected, such as in the metabolism disorders mentioned above. Jane needs to manage and plan the use of her body's flexibility over time to maximize her healthspan.

To use a comparative example from everyday life, think about this: when extra work piles up, Jane will have various options to deal with the situation. We believe she should not interrupt her regular sleep patterns if possible because sleep patterns are deeply embedded evolutionarily in her physiology. Therefore, trying to change them challenges many of her core systems and functions that are deeply automated to coordinate with the day-night cycle.[21]

Conversely, consistent sleep patterns in line with the evolution of core systems keep their environment consistent and reliable and actually allow her to meet daily challenges more effectively and with less stress. She can actually take on more new activities or problems than she could if she were constantly challenged by late nights or unmanaged dietary habits; after all, many aspects of digestion are also directly linked to core systems like endocrine functioning (such as fat storage) or even the day-night cycle.

All systems of the body sense their environments, change, and adjust to them. Even if a sensed change is due to declining functional demand from a related system, we believe it can result in the lowering of *their* functions as well. There may be no reason to continue producing a given product—or keeping a function at a given level—if it is no longer needed. For example, impaired heart function can lead to a lowering of the functional capacity of nearly all systems, since the resource delivery and demands they are used to providing have been altered. This is why there are so many disease states related to each other: the body is an ecosystem of intelligent groups and systems, and if one group is compromised, other groups may also be affected depending on the person's constitution or other factors. Finally, regarding core systems, loss of all function in one—like an organ—can lead to total system failure (death) or at least severely affected health. This is not the case with loss of function in a joint or even in an entire limb.

To return to Jane's company for an example, if the sales department can no longer sell the product, the company needs to change and may downsize not only sales but also production and possibly other core departments. On the other hand, the sales department itself may be quite flexible as to size, and if short-term fluctuations in demand occur, it might not demand that the core departments change.

Modern Problems

We believe the ramifications of the mismatch between our modern environment and our evolutionary past will continue to unfold as people growing up with the modern challenges we spoke of experience even more sicknesses at younger ages. It has taken a long time for many problems to emerge because the human body has great intelligence, flexibility, and repair potential, especially in its younger years. But we believe that, to some extent, these modern challenges are using flex potential early on that will be needed as the population ages.

We are addressing stress and the lack of the physical activities as the primary target for Jane's program, which we present in Chapter 6. The first one challenges her flexibility capacity to an excessive degree, and the second challenges it with a lack of use. Both challenge some core systems and some flexible systems.

Besides the increase in various chronic problems we see—such as metabolic disorder, heart disease, or cancer—the population will also be more susceptible to related problems, even things like epidemic-like events as internal environments, communication, and flexibility potential deteriorate.

Jane is younger than many people experiencing the increase of metabolic disorder, diabetes, and obesity, but diabetes runs in her family, and she sees what is coming and is looking for answers. If she understands that her propensity to gain weight or get stressed out has evolutionary roots, she can at least begin to look at things in a different light. While it seems modern high-stress, quickly changing environments and lifestyles are unavoidable, it is important to understand that the dynamics include not just the quantity but also the speed of change demanded. Therefore, we don't necessarily look at modern environmental demands as bad but rather as something that needs to be understood as an adjustment issue, which takes time and varies from person to person. This is another reason we need a wide-scope, long-term framework that can encompass many different individualized health and fitness needs.

Of course, we all need to make physical demands on our bodies, which is the purpose of Jane's workouts. But we also need to manage the demands we encounter—and even create them for ourselves. We need a framework for *managed change*, which is the purpose of our upcoming discussion on ideas for Jane's healthspan.

For example, trying to process information too quickly or simply too much information at a time—too much mental work—can be stressful. Too many problems to solve too quickly from too many sources in our high-information society is a problem. But there are timelines to stress as well, which can be managed through planning. Taking on unattainable goals or too many long-term projects can create stress, as can the short-term information overload of something more immediate. But if we understand that feeling stress under the above circumstances is evolutionarily normal, we can try to manage the incoming information and, therefore, the stress level. We will address managing our incoming information by creating a mental framework for it later in this book, but first, we'll look at managing Jane's fitness activities.

Fitness as an Environmental Demand

We have used the general term "environmental demands" simply because it is well-known in biology that the environment induces biological changes in all living things.[22] Therefore, looking at our world in terms of an environment in this way can remind us to be aware that on a moment-to-moment basis, everything we see, do, or intend to do—including work, diet, sleep, daily activities, and even our fitness programs—induce internal changes and affect our healthspan. These are all part of the environment within which the body will continually attempt to change itself to perform optimally.

We look at Jane's fitness programs as an intentionally formulated part of her environment with which her body aligns itself and a part of the time she has set aside to benefit her health. They are an intentional challenge she puts herself through, and as manager of her life, she needs to choose the ones that fit her future goals the best. When Jane played basketball in college, a managed framework was used to encompass many different levels, from planning whole seasons down to a single day's practice session. Practice was set up to simulate future demands: the expected future scenarios in an actual game or event. This pushed each player individually within the context of team-work to respond in a way that improved function and efficiency based on what is perceived to be coming in the future.

With enough repeated demand of given activities, the body will plan for the fact that this activity is likely to continue, and physical changes will be made to improve efficiency in that area. When practicing free throws and also with the team as a unit, Jane's body was planning ahead: her related systems and their memory changed. We want Jane to consider such practice time in sports as similar to the fitness programs in her life today: a formulated demand thought to be helpful for her future goals. We want Jane to take on the role of the coach and general *manager* for the whole season or more.

When we say that Jane's body plans ahead based on her intentions and activity, we can look at marathon runners or weightlifters as examples. We can clearly see that a body shape develops corresponding to optimizing that activity: lifting weights with certain muscles leads to increased capacity for that activity, including enlarged muscles. Runners, on the other hand, often need to do other activities, such as some weightlifting, or they will drop upper body mass based on that activity. Whatever the demand is from the environment, so to speak, our entire body will try to respond as best it can.

Another aspect of the term *environmental demand* is that it also implies inclusion of future situations in the management of life's changes. The body makes changes when enough experience or repetition has occurred for given systems to assume it will continue into the future.

We believe future events should be managed and planned for when formulating fitness programs, even factors like having a child, getting a new job, being relocated, or retiring. The body evolved to adjust itself for many environmental changes and cycles, like day and night (of course), but also for long-term cycles, such as seasons and stages of life. By formulating an intended evolution framework to include one's entire healthspan, the body can plan for short-and long-term goals, and it will use its flexibility capacity accordingly.

Jane's Fitness Today

Sports and fitness have been a part of human societies for thousands of years, and they are important in most cultures. Today, there are many ideas as to what it is to be *fit*, but *fitness* is generally associated with being in a "healthy physical condition" or having a "fit look," as defined by popular culture. Fitness has also become closely associated with sports, usually involving competition to display some form of specialized performance. The details of exercise physiology in relation to specialized performance or the look of the body have been studied in great detail over the years, and many programs have been designed from these details. Physical activities are important to staying healthy, yet in our modern world, we use them less and less in our normal, everyday lives. Therefore, efficient fitness programs are more important today than ever before.

A typical fitness program for someone like Jane often focuses on increasing heart rate and overall metabolic rates in order to burn calories that she has recently eaten—and, hopefully, her extra fat. This is often done by placing demands on various (usually large) muscles through any number of activities and repeating these demands enough times per week to burn calories and maintain or build muscle mass.

For example, Jane has recently tried activities that use large muscles to burn a lot of calories as well as build up those muscles so they will burn calories during the day, even when she isn't working out. We want Jane to use a managed approach to review these and other activities to try to optimize what she is doing based on her goals. We feel a split can occur between fitness and long-term health because exercise is often separated from everyday activity.

Currently, Jane usually sees exercise as something rather stressful or even miserable, and she wants to get it done as quickly as possible and move on with the rest of her day. We want Jane's fitness programs or activities to also become more integrated into her everyday life when possible; a framework to maximize her healthspan includes embedding parts of her routine into her normal day. We also want her to enjoy what she is doing and make sure her fitness activities lead to progress towards her long-term goals. We will speak more about the importance of playfulness and enjoyment later.

With respect to her latest activities above, let's look at the physiological demands of repeatedly using her large muscles to burn calories. We could say the immediate demand on her body during the workout is for energy or calories for those muscles. Then, if repeated over time, the muscle cells and tissues will begin to change and get larger. More protein will be demanded of the other systems (digestive, liver, etc.) to build more muscle. The new muscle will need to be maintained by the heart, lungs, and other systems. While Jane doesn't necessarily want larger muscles just for the sake of having them, this is a goal because larger muscles and higher metabolism rates burn more calories.

This oft-used high-metabolism, calorie-burning model is a limited view in the context of Jane's situation and the overall human condition, in our opinion. We are also skeptical that burning calories by building the large muscles will necessarily lead to even her medium-term goal of losing weight, especially in Jane's current situation. Furthermore, looking at the larger picture, we can see that larger muscles, once built, will also need to be maintained.

Taking Jane's house as an analogy, if she expands or adds on to the current one, it is not just a matter of adding another room with the function of extra space, although that is the intent. During the process, systems such as water and electric need to be upgraded in various ways, and going forward, maintenance costs in many forms have increased. The new space needs to be heated or air conditioned, and larger floor and wall space (which requires cleaning, painting, and even higher taxes) all add to costs and maintenance effort going forward. Jane wants to make sure to add space and spend the money where she really needs it, where there is a functional need; in other words, it wouldn't make sense for Jane to add a room to her house that she doesn't really need.

The physiological responses Jane notices when she places demands on her large muscles are a hunger response for more calories for fuel, protein to build muscles up, and various changes related to a higher metabolism. Of course, this puts demands on all her related systems; there is a whole chain of effects and changes, and any change has costs in energy and flexibility. Like the larger home, being larger means spending more; Jane will be hungrier, needing to take in more calories to maintain the structure and higher metabolism rate. Furthermore, muscles learn a task and get better at it over time to save energy and resources, resulting in a plateau effect. This can lead to the need to increase a workout's intensity for continued results. Over time, Jane may need to lift more and need to accelerate her workouts, partly because it isn't really part of her normal lifestyle.

With the high caloric intake in today's modern societies—and the associated sedentary lifestyles—it is understandable that maximum calorie-burning activities or programs have become a good short-term answer. Essentially, today's lifestyle has created a need for time-efficient activities that can burn the calories we are accustomed to taking in, but in a relatively short time. This pattern (a lack of activity followed by ramped-up metabolism), from the intended evolution point of view, can send contrary signals to the body that certain functions aren't normally needed, followed by needing them in a big way but on a short-term basis. In this way, like stop-and-go traffic, Jane is on the accelerator and then brakes, on and off, as she goes through life. This is inefficient and can create undue wear and tear as well as be a very difficult way to lose weight for some people because these types of activities lead to an increased appetite, which can be miserable to try to fight.

If Jane is not careful, too much demand, too little, or both on her various systems will lead to stressing her internal flexibility capacity as her body continually attempts adjustments to fit the conflicting level of activity and caloric intake. There is nothing wrong with high-calorie burn and muscle building if Jane wants or needs it; this was a fine framework for her college basketball days because performance was a primary goal, both short- and mid-term. But for her lifestyle today, this is similar to her owning an expensive race car, paying for high performance when she really just needs something to get her to work. She is spending too much on maintenance and gas for something she doesn't really need.

We are not worried about Jane's arm and leg muscles responding or wearing out, as they are flexible and meant to change relatively quickly and often to meet differing demand levels. But we believe there are downsides to high-metabolism, high-burn types of activities because they often entail a significant amount of stress on other parts of the body, using flexibility that will be important later in life. The current movement toward the mega-workout, distance running, or ultra-high demands of professional type sports challenges the flex capacity of many functions, including core functions (like the heart) in an unneeded way.[23]

Intended Evolution Fitness

Using our ideas to review her activities, Jane reports that her current short-term goal is to burn calories—and hopefully fat. When pressed for her long-term goals, she says she wants to lose weight and, finally, be healthy in the long run. So, we will call her mid-term goal losing weight and her long-term goal to be healthy, which, according to Jane, is also a primary goal. Using these short-, medium-, and long-term goals, we will look at what she has been doing so far according to intended evolution, and then, in Chapter 6, we'll give her some recommendations on using it. We want Jane to be the "general manager" of her life, so to speak, setting goals and managing her life from the top down. Her short-term activities should provide *cumulative directional progress* toward her future goals, including lifelong good health and a long healthspan.

Using the intended evolution framework, we want Jane to use a wide-scope view of who she is and what she is really trying to achieve in the future and then decide which exercise routines she can use to best match what she wants. Physical activities or workouts get their value from the goals, long- and short-term, that they are intended to achieve and what it takes to get there. One reason Jane wants to lose weight is to look better, but she is also aware that in her case losing some weight would be beneficial for her health. An activity aiming for a certain look may be the goal, or it may be a result and not necessarily a goal in itself.

Of course, there is nothing wrong with being motivated to achieve a certain look, performance metrics, or even high remodel, such as trying to compete in sports or fitness like she did in college. But using the intended evolution framework, the first step in addressing the *how* to get somewhere is by simply asking *why* are we doing a given activity: what is the goal, and how does it fit into the big picture? Does Jane *want* to have a certain look? To be able to run very fast? To run or cycle long distances, or lift a lot of weight? Or, is she using these activities for other purposes? Her muscles probably have no problem keeping up, but what about the other systems? Is a high-caloric intake, high-metabolism lifestyle right for Jane at this point in her life?

We know different body types result from different activities, such as distance runners compared to weightlifters, swimmers, or even sprinters. Jane's body is very intelligent and, although slower than her college days, will try to change itself based on what she does, so any activity needs to be taken in a context with her goals in mind. In Jane's case, at this point in her life, she really wants to lose some weight (to both look and feel better) and generally stay as healthy as possible to attain the longest possible health-span.

Of course, common sense tells her that becoming overweight weakens many functions and leads to poor health, and everyone knows you can't just do nothing, since that quickens the unwanted results. Jane's previous activities, and those of millions of other people, were essentially meant to build and maintain increased muscle mass through high-calorie, high-burn metabolism programs, which obviously have many benefits compared to lack of activity.

Let's look at how some of Jane's internal systems and metabolism were affected when she started her mega-workout:

1.) Jane's activities used her large muscles, which in turn burned calories.

2.) The digestive system tried to replace the calories burned, and therefore, Jane got hungrier and tended to eat more.

3.) Repeated demands on her muscles signaled her body to build and maintain more muscle mass, which also led to a higher caloric intake, preferentially for protein.

Jane could easily get bigger, not smaller, if she is not careful to fight her craving for food, which she often reports as difficult to do. Furthermore, she will need to maintain her new larger and higher metabolism rate, again with greater food intake. This also requires other metabolic activities to break it down, use it, and dispose of the waste.

We believe that this activity means Jane's body was using its flex capacity, including core metabolic systems, in order to make all the changes needed to build muscle and maintain a higher metabolism level. This is spending flex capacity for something she may or may not need given her goals.

Furthermore, whenever Jane took a break from her rigorous routine, her body tended to react accordingly over time, again using flex capacity to change. In other words, as her activity level went down, her body used its ability to change in order to reverse the buildup of her muscles. It does this because it is highly intelligent and thrifty; maintaining more than is needed was historically expensive and inefficient and was selected against in her evolution. Jane can end up on a hamster wheel, so to speak, if she's not careful. Maintaining muscle or any tissue that isn't needed is a waste of the body's resources, including the flexibility potential it needs for a long healthspan.

One example of using the body's flex capacity upfront is the extreme remodeling demands of some professional sports we see today (although recently, even some fitness programs are copying this model). Besides the obvious wear and tear that can come with excessive high-burn, high-impact activities (which can inhibit needed functions going forward), other core system troubles, such as heart health,[10] are also emerging from these types of high-performance activities. We believe this is because some of the body's limited capacity for flexibility is being "front-loaded," so to speak, and that many systems can lose their flexibility with too much demand for change from these types of activities.

This is like a driver constantly accelerating and putting on the brakes versus using a smoother driving experience. You have higher wear and tear on brakes and many other parts, and you have to use more energy in the process. You can achieve a smoother driving experience by looking further down the road and knowing where you are and where you are going, taking action at the right time. Perhaps you should plan out the trip in advance, use the freeway or a route with fewer stops, or even take fewer trips in the first place, making your vehicle last longer.

Chapter 4

HEALTHSPAN STRATEGIES

In this chapter, we will discuss some of the ways the evolution of living things can help us understand our healthspan potential and some general ideas or strategies that can help Jane manage hers. As we've said, matching her evolutionary past with where she wants to go can help her decide "what type of car to drive," so to speak—which body is best for the most efficient ride and maximum healthspan. To discuss longevity, we will assume that a long *functional lifespan* (i.e., a long healthspan) is a valid goal for Jane and then look at a couple of examples from nature from which she can borrow.

Stable Environments

This longevity strategy is based on populations with long healthspans in the world today that can be found in areas where life is simple and moves forward in an "old-world," very predictable way. We see this in certain fishing or farming villages in Japan or other areas of the world known for longevity. The key here is the *consistency* and *predictability* of environmental signals, requiring few behavioral or physical changes. People specialize to fit a lifestyle and diet in line with their evolution, and there is little surprising or unexpected change needed going forward in their lives: they know where they are going and what they will be doing in the future. As we noted earlier, not only is this is the opposite of what causes mental overload and stress, but it also leads to less demand for internal physical change. We also want to note that this lifestyle seems quite contrary to much of the high-stimulation, "experience as much as you can, as fast as you can" culture we often see today.

Another aspect of this example is that the body tends to optimize itself during development, and little change is needed after that. During the early years of life, the body gets better and better at what is required of it to deal with its environment. At the same time, when the environment does not change much, one's body becomes efficient at what is actually needed and by what systems. Furthermore, the body generally doesn't need to keep a wide range of flexibility capacity available but rather uses flexibility potential for a longer life in the same consistent direction. *This essentially leads to regularity and a stable routine with few surprises, which is important for following long-term plans and reaching goals.*

Like these societies, Jane can try to keep her environment as stable and predictable as possible and know where she is going. The idea here is to use information, activities, and patterns that her body has evolved to use in an amount and way that helps her reach her goals. We see talk of this strategy beginning to make a comeback in some areas in recent years with a steady movement toward "slow food," whole foods, local organic farming, calmer lifestyles, and other "back to basics" activities. We will not deal with actual dietary information in this book, although we feel eating foods that we evolved to eat at the times we evolved to eat them saves the body from spending flex capacity on digestive adjustments. We do believe modern diets and living conditions can be a big problem today and into the future as compounds we didn't evolve with proliferate. Ultimately it is our individual cells that evolved to utilize certain nutrients over evolutionary history and we believe this should be a guide in deciding what they should be subjected to.

With a life of low stress and very few surprises, necessary use of flexibility (or remodeling) is kept to a minimum, and one can use energy and flex capacity for a longer, relatively change-free life. In this strategy, Jane would still use all of the evolutionarily important available functions in her body in a consistent, balanced manner—but not so as to wear them out. Essentially, our bodies evolved like a well-honed tool, not unlike the perfect-sized wrench or screwdriver, for the task of dealing with those environments. The human body is our tool and is best used for the purposes for which it evolved, so we don't want to try to alter it too much. Jane doesn't want her tool to sit and rust, but she also doesn't want too much wear and tear; she wants stable, predictable usage patterns within normal capacity limits.

Of course, Jane can't go back to everything her ancestors did, but she *can* recognize and use aspects of them in her modern life. For example, she can use basic historical eating and sleeping patterns as the backdrop for her life to help augment consistency and regularity in her activities. She can also use evolutionary environmental signals in the visualizations she does (see Chapter 5). Many lifeforms on earth whose environments are relatively stable—certain trees, sea life, or low-activity animals like lobsters or turtles—have the kind of lifestyle that fulfills the evolutionary history of that given organism. They experience very stable conditions with little change and have evolved to deal with the limited challenges they *do* face very well. Essentially, they rarely use flex capacity and energy for new environmental challenges, but rather, it is used for a longer lifespan.

While this strategy seems to go against our point that modern environments are changing faster and faster, we still want Jane to use aspects of this strategy for her core systems and use her more flexible systems to deal with change.

Long Lifespan as an Environmental Demand

Another strategy Jane can copy from the natural world is to live within a set of environmental demands that call for long life for a purpose deemed important for survival. Longer lifespans allow for more varied strategies of survival by living long enough to utilize longer-term patterns in nature. Seasonal patterns, for example, create a niche for employing strategies such as hibernation or migration that give those able to utilize them an advantage for some niches versus shorter-lived organisms. When animals began to recognize and utilize such long-term patterns, we believe it created (environmental) demands on their internal systems to operate longer, tending to change and stretch out their functional lifespans.[24] Essentially, the perception of an advantage to living longer leads the body's systems to use flex capacity to reach that goal, rather than spending it in other areas.

As for Jane, her choices and actions on a day-to-day basis can be coordinated into a long healthspan strategy by planning important events far into the future. She can essentially create demands in the form of certain future goals, and her internal systems will also plan for a longer life. We address this concept more fully in the next chapter and then specifically in Chapter 6, with visualizations designed for Jane to plan a long life that her health and fitness activities should fit within. With this strategy, energy and flexibility are directed for the purpose of living longer in order to achieve important goals, which evidence suggests can increase longevity and reduce signs of aging.[25]

In one of the studies cited, even such things as having long-term business goals can keep one healthier and increase longevity. Near death, there is evidence the intention to wait for an important event like a loved one's arrival or even a birthday milestone can affect the time of death.[26] One anecdote we find very interesting is a well-known story: our early presidents Thomas Jefferson and John Adams, while political adversaries at times, kept in contact late in life and badly wanted to see our country's fiftieth birthday. Although in poor health, they both made it, dying on the same day: July 4, 1826.

Consider the story of Albert Brown, an American soldier during World War II:

> Following the Bataan Death March, Brown endured a three-year imprisonment in a Japanese POW camp from 1942 until he was liberated in the middle of September 1945. He ate nothing but rice while in the camp. Brown became afflicted with more than twelve diseases while in the camp, including dengue fever, malaria, and dysentery. He also suffered a broken neck and back. He was released from the camp when he was 40 years old. He was nearly blind from maltreatment and had lost more than eighty pounds, then weighing less than one hundred pounds. A doctor told Brown that he would not live to be 50 years old due to the extent of his injuries. However, he lived to be 105 years old.[27]

We not only have amazing and untapped mental capabilities to affect our own bodies and health, but when focused on important goals going forward, the physical body can respond in ways not yet fully appreciated in today's world. Anecdotal cases like Jefferson and Adams waiting for a future date to die or Albert Brown's incredible physical flexibility tend to be dismissed because they are "unscientific." But many amazing events of human potential cannot be tested in a lab, and we believe that a common thread for many such examples of human potential is the will to live and the intention to make it happen. We can use these basic aspects ourselves—which include our own innate internal medicine—in a planned and systematic way to improve our health and lives going forward.

Henry Ford is credited with saying, "Whether you think you can, or you think you cannot, you're right."

The Constant Emergency Strategy

Of course, there are many "strategies" used for survival (and we are generalizing in our presentation here), and we can use knowledge about evolution to help us with our health. The previous two strategies are ones we can incorporate into our lives and fitness programs, and we believe them to be very helpful. We also want to include another example, something we want Jane to avoid in the long term.

There are also many niches that developed when environmental conditions called for rapid change or, sometimes, short-term opportunities that might end quickly. Some organisms tended to focus on short-term patterns to meet those demands and take advantage of those niches, resulting in a lifespan focused on the short term, for example, or reproducing quickly during a short period of opportunity. A short lifespan can also make a lot of sense in order to take full advantage of certain conditions—after a rain or a winter thaw that won't last long, for instance.

We might draw parallels here to the "live fast and die young" slogan or lifestyle some embrace. When one believes everything important needs to happen quickly and the long term may not happen, there is little reason for the body to plan for a long healthspan. This mindset and lack of long-term planning can also lead to an uncertain future and lots of surprises, as we will see.

The intelligent human body will also adjust to short-term demands if need be, regardless of long-term implications like lifespan. In emergency situations, the body can automatically sacrifice the long-term for a short-term urgency, such as during starvation, when the body—and even cells—will break down areas not currently critical in favor of survival functions.[28] In this case, the signal from the external environment says there might not be a long term without quick change now. This is not conducive to long-term health, but it is advantageous evolutionarily in certain cases—one the body is willing to perform to survive a current crisis. We want to avoid current crises when possible, not create them. Planning for the future essentially mitigates short-term uncertainty and crisis in favor of a smoother transition to the future.

We especially don't want Jane to impose this strategy on her core systems at this point in her life because it is an example of using flex capacity "up front," so to speak. We believe that extreme remodel activities can signal the body to use its flexibility and resources now, whereas future goals, such as longevity, are not a high priority. We sometimes see motivational focus, or power techniques, that tend to use this strategy. There is nothing wrong with any of these techniques in general, but they are best used in a long-term context or during high-flexibility stages in life rather than as a regular strategy throughout life.

Therefore, we believe that while extremely demanding high-remodel fitness may get you a certain look or high performance short-term, it could also shorten your health-span and lifespan.

This should lead us to question whether attitudes like "more is always better" or "work hard, play hard" always make sense. Are they simply an attempt to motivate ourselves over and over for the short term? We want Jane to manage her situation within her long-term framework because her mega-workout can have a similar—but of course, not as severe—effect as the "constant emergency" strategy above if she's not careful. The signal to Jane's body says to use its flex capacity (which includes future healing potential) to build her a larger body and a higher metabolism rate, triggering greater demands on her cardiovascular, digestive, endocrine, and other functions. If these demands are too high, they can be counterproductive going forward.

Using our framework, at this point in her life, Jane needs smoother, more consistent activities and a lifestyle that fits her long-term goals for maximum healthspan. Constantly reacting in the short term, such as working out extra after gaining five pounds, is not unlike running her car in a high-maintenance "stop and go fashion" as opposed to having a longer, smoother, more efficient ride. Jane can create many demands for her body on a day-to-day basis that keep her healthy and result in cumulative directional progress towards her long-term goals. In this way, her workouts or fitness programs aren't seen as separate from the rest of her day but rather as part of her framework, with her long-term goals at the top (primary).

Jane can manage her activities and limit the constant upsizing, downsizing, and maintenance of unneeded function when possible, reducing the cost in flexibility of her body's systems going forward.

Sports and Long-Term Frameworks

Pertaining to the previous discussion about professional sports and high-intensity workout regimes, we want to clarify that we are not saying these are "bad" or that they always send signals to shorten one's life. There are many different body types and potentials among different people, and depending on where they are in their lives, use of future flex potential from a given activity will vary. For example, the body naturally has more potential remodel (flexibility) capacity when younger, and it makes sense that performance activities take place at certain times in one's lifespan.

However, planning properly for a professional sports career, for example, including when it is ending, can be highly beneficial to the professional athlete in helping him or her limit lost flexibility going forward. This is not unlike the way an astronaut prepares for the physiological demands of weightlessness for his or her upcoming trip but also plans for the needed adjustment period upon return. This is especially the case when managing the end of an athlete's professional sports stage. We believe there needs to an awareness that when we *do* build for high-demand sports, there will be a need to return to baseline when that part of our lives is finished. A long-term plan would dictate keeping the high-functioning levels they attained that make sense for their healthspan framework, such as hand-eye coordination or balance skills. However, for other factors, such as muscle mass for certain strength usages, a gradually managed deceleration from peak performance to normal life in a well-planned way can help to avoid undue health problems later in life.

In general, we need to manage our bodies as intelligently and efficiently as possible and adjust when needed. At times, former athletes simply try to maintain their previous bodies through the same—although less intense—techniques as before. Attempting to continue a high-level use of flexibility potential for unneeded functions can be unhelpful for or hinder long-term goals once a new part of life begins. Fitting all the different parts of one's life into one framework with him or her as the managing director helps individualize health and fitness goals and programs.

Long-Distance Travelers: A Long Healthspan

Finally, we want to discuss the concept mentioned earlier of having a good level of proficiency in core life functions for the entire lifespan. Early in life, long-term health versus short-term wants and needs are blurred, and this is probably for good evolutionary reasons. Part of the point of early life is to use flexibility in order to test and discover how to best fit into the surrounding environment. But as we grow, especially as modern humans, being aware of long-term goals is very helpful in attempting to optimize the use of our flex potential going forward.

Therefore, when formulating a health and fitness strategy, taking longer-term plans (even the entire lifespan) into account makes sense. We want as much of Jane's life, including her fitness programs, to create cumulative progress towards her goal of keeping her needed functions in good working order for as long as possible.

Jane can take parts from both of the previously discussed longevity strategies to create and manage a framework to try and minimize the things that signal shorter lifespan—those that use her flex capacity unnecessarily and maximize signals for a long life. We could look at this as "riding the line of optimal use" of a given body: not too much function demand upfront—limited stress and flexibility use—but still enough demand to keep important functions that the body will need well into her planned future.

From strategy one, we want to retain consistency and predictability for our core evolutionary functions when possible by not demanding too much quick change. As we've mentioned, what we call core functions and structures are stable and relatively inflexible simply because there was evolutionarily little challenge and demand for change.

One example of a challenge to core functions in today's world is working late at night—or all night—and trying to adjust with erratic sleep patterns or sleeping during the day. This challenges a basic environmental pattern we evolved to follow at the core levels of much of our physiology. Therefore, trying to change this very predictable and stable pattern of behavior from our evolution can negatively affect long-term health. According to our framework, any erratic patterns of behavior related to core functions, such as sleeping or eating at inconsistent or odd times, are not conducive to long-term health because related physiological functions are (evolutionarily) deeply tied to their cycles and did not evolve to change much. When possible, related activities should be fit into the basic day-night cycle of life and other patterns with long evolutionary history.

We know Jane can't just move to a fishing village to protect her core functions, but she *can* use the principles from strategy one above (consistency) to manage her core functions as she also draws from strategy two (interfacing with environmental factors and having goals that demand a long life). Essentially, strategy two is engaging in activities with long feedback cycles where the brain organizes information based on longer cycles, and the subconscious will push her systems towards longevity (see the next chapter).

Jane can maintain and protect core functions and create demands that direct her flex capacity to be used for a long life by using her intelligence. By planning for a long life, the cycles, like the ones discussed, as well as her other behaviors, will take on longer-term context and meaning, as we will see in the next chapter.

Chapter 5

MIND-BODY FITNESS AND MEDICINE

In any evolutionary theory, both what an organism is currently (its DNA, physical attributes, abilities, etc.) and its environment are important factors in what Darwin called "the struggle for life." According to intended evolution, our perceptions and intentions and their effect on our internal systems are also very important to evolution as well as changes in our bodies during this lifetime.

As we have said, Jane begins her interactions—or "struggle"—based on her DNA blueprint, but her perceptions and intelligence allow her to make choices about how she uses it. Therefore, her unique human intelligence affords her great flexibility to employ strategies with which to best use her DNA blueprint to benefit her in this lifetime.

As any sports team knows, during the game, intelligent adjustments must constantly be made because each game, like our environment, is always changing—you don't just keep doing things that obviously aren't working. Similarly, Jane can flexibly manage her activities and make adjustments as life changes and new information comes in.

Much of our discussion on flexibility has been about physical change in our bodies, which we have noted is also intelligent at the local level, but in this chapter, we will deal with Jane's most important source of flexibility: her highly evolved mental capacities.

Change and the Environment

It is well documented that organisms are able to change—sometimes dramatically—based on changes in their environments.[29] For example, a school of clownfish is always built into a hierarchy with a female fish at the top. When she dies, the most dominant male changes sex and takes her place. There are many other dramatic examples of change, including organisms that have different shapes, sizes, and colors depending on what type of environment they develop in. The study of developmental biology reveals many interesting examples of this type in which the environment "induces" an organism to change form, color, or behavior.

According to intended evolution, organisms intelligently interface with the environment via their perceptions, which can therefore be seen as a "cause" of internal changes. Historically, the idea that all life forms (including our own internal cells) are intelligent and perceive things is not normally included in the study of environmental effects or biology in general. But what we are saying in regards to intended evolution is not that an organism understands its internal workings (such as options for shape or color) but rather, like all living things, that its internal systems have also evolved to act in certain ways depending on what they perceive.

This is similar to the situation we mentioned earlier—Jane building muscle in her fitness classes—when her internal intelligence perceives the need to change, her muscles will get larger or smaller automatically based on what Jane does. Notice we say larger *or* smaller; lack of use results in fewer resources going toward a given function (in this case, muscle size). Lack of challenge—such as when astronauts go to space or a person is confined to bed for long periods of time—can create an environment where not only muscle but bone or even heart mass are shed.[30]

Starting fitness classes or going to outer space are both actually "demands for change" based on a change in various demand levels in the new environment. We don't necessarily look at the resulting changes as bad or good in themselves but rather as natural adjustments made by our intelligent bodies. Of course, overuse or damage of internal systems can create unwanted change as well—like when joints, tissues, or cells are challenged too severely and do not return to their original state (lung cells in smokers, for example).

Notice that here we aren't *telling* our bodies to do all these things, but each system does what it evolved to do in its own way to optimally fit the environment the person is in. What we do and what we perceive filter down to a given cell or system based on how communication patterns evolved and are part of the environment they react to.

Awareness and Information Sharing

Jane changes based on her perceptions and her physical activities within her environment. As discussed earlier, we don't really need to view Jane's mental and physical aspects as separate (except for the sake of discussion) but rather as part of each other. In our view, one purpose of the nervous system and the brain is sharing information between all the internal living systems in order for them to act as one unit: Jane's sense of self. More generally, and important to health, is that Jane's internal cells and systems are part of a communication system that perceives Jane's world and also affects the way Jane perceives the world.

Jane's mental clarity in interfacing with her external environment is obviously very important; based on the intended evolution framework, her mental functions are influenced by the health of her internal life. When Jane has an internal problem, it can result in the direction of more resources and attention to that local area. If the internal trouble is large enough, a lessening or disruption can affect her ability to perform mental functions. A simple example is when time off and downtime is needed because she is ill or otherwise not feeling well. This is a natural result of her internal systems needing more energy, leaving less to face external situations. In the same way, Jane's perceptions can affect her internal systems, such as when she gets scared or becomes angry.[31] Information and research related to the above discussion are essentially what we believe helps explain and will continue to drive the mind-body paradigm shift going forward, including other areas of health as well. Aspects of Jane's mind interface with both the internal communication of her body as well as with her external world.

Jane's company is again a simple analogy. There are many employees and department managers that share information with each other internally to produce their product—and those who communicate with the outside such as sales, customer relations, or delivery—but the company is also managed as a single unit. In large companies, upper-level managers often have little to no idea of the small details in many departments; they are concerned with major activities and decisions about the overall direction the company is going. Jane and other managers in her company have to balance internal and external factors by paying attention to which products they can sell *and also* making sure they can produce and deliver them.

This last point is a basic aspect of the mind-body paradigm: it can be very helpful for Jane to pay attention to her internal systems as well as her external surroundings. We recommend that she monitor her body and how it feels when working out at the gym rather than listening to or watching the news during her fitness activities, for example. This is a basic mind-body premise and essentially brings the body's awareness and intelligence back to what is happening in the moment, which increases internal communication and the effectiveness of the activity.

Jane's Highly Evolved (Human) Intelligence

The intelligent aspects of organisms have become more and more powerful and important with the greater complexity of life, although ultimately driven by the survival instinct. Clearly, intelligence is a big evolutionary advantage, and it makes sense that it has generally increased over time. Although we think of all lifeforms exhibiting intelligence using the term broadly, advanced humans evolved amazing abilities related to recognizing, processing, saving, and using information. Jane's ancestors (and societies in general) have become more able to change their environments, reducing many demands on their bodies to carry out many previously needed functions. We call this ability to change the environment "strategic use of the environment," and it even includes things like living in caves, making nests, making and using tools, and especially advanced communication and interaction with others. All of these things require complex actions, and as they became more elaborate over time, they make intelligence even more useful and, therefore, an evolutionary advantage.

Fast-forward to modern humans and our increase in processing power, which brought us the powerful ability to picture things and "run scenarios" in our minds. In short, the ability to hold, compare, or process enough information (including from memory) resulted in a scenario-running ability, which was a huge evolutionary advantage. This is so because for any given situation—such as when one needs to escape a predator—only one choice is made (run, fight, climb, etc.); we cannot try them all at once nor have the chance to fail and try another. But running scenarios allows for multiple "virtual actions" for a given situation, from which the perceived best outcome can be chosen. Of course, much of this process "runs in the background," so to speak, and it is often subconscious to some extent.

Very important to the mind-body concept and the basis of the intended evolution framework is that this process also plays out over time based not only on the present moment but also on what is intended in the future. As information comes in and events unfold, scenarios or possibilities are sorted and evaluated based on what we intend to do. Our unconscious mind is always "thinking ahead" and formulating future action scenarios based on our past experiences (memory), what is happening now, and what we plan and intend to do in the future. This is a very important understanding for the future of the mind-body paradigm, as is the earlier discussion that different levels of intelligence (including unconscious) are meant to be working on important upcoming events. Clearing one's mind to reduce stress is being found to be very beneficial of course, but we need to understand that having many possible upcoming events, possibilities, or challenges means the different layers of our intelligence will naturally tend to work on them. This makes managing our futures very valuable in reaching and sustaining this goal.

Planning

Planning is essentially "projecting," or estimating, future outcomes; when done accurately, it alleviates the stress of surprise or uncertainty in the present and going forward. Jane tends to be a very organized person (she has plans she sticks with), which automatically tends to mitigate some of her stress. Because stress can occur due to unexpected or surprising information in the environment, her ability to plan ahead and organize her life to fit her future plans is an important tool she already tends to use.

Planning also allows better management of the resources you have: you waste less time and effort—and use fewer resources—when you know where you're going and what you'll be doing in the future. We tend to take the ability to plan our future for granted, but it is actually a complex and important evolutionary tool and the basis of the intended evolution framework.

To discuss this further, we want to speak briefly about some aspects of the information we perceive in our environment. The very nature of information is a "pattern" that repeats and can therefore be used to make projections or estimates about the future. For example, the very reliable day-night cycle we mentioned before has been used throughout evolution to develop useful strategies for things such as a finding food or hiding when predators are likely present. Even something simple, like always knowing the exact location of a safe hiding spot, is an example of reliability of information that allows for a good plan. For Jane, her paycheck is very steady and reliable, and she extrapolates that information to predict her future income, allowing behavior and planning that wouldn't otherwise be possible (an apartment lease or car loan, for example).

Furthermore, as one can imagine, any such longer information patterns that allow projections or estimates further away from us in time (the future) and space (physical distance) are also very valuable. When survival is on the line, the further one can see, the further ahead the plan is made and the bigger the advantage for survival chances. For example, it is advantageous when animals can recognize a predator further away (distance) or when the weather will soon turn cold for winter (time).

According to Intended Evolution, larger and larger "patterns" of information were recognized and able to be used as evolution of intelligence progressed. For example, when day-to-day weather was able to be taken in the context of seasons, it gave it greater meaning: certain animals could determine when winter was coming and therefore knew that colder weather would soon arrive on a daily basis, not just as a one-time event. What we think of as "timelines" are information patterns of different lengths of time in our memory, and longer timelines allow us to make plans further into the future. Our brains process information patterns based on past (memory), present (present perceptions), and future (plans), all in relation to each other, and among other things, longer timelines allow more efficient responses to what is coming. They tend to be very useful in reducing surprises and stress in the present and enhanced survival during evolution. Jane knows that often, the longer the timeline (further into the future) she uses to plan for upcoming deadlines at work, the less stress she has because her life tends to unfold as expected.

One interesting aspect of timelines was touched on earlier: our subconscious runs off not only our memories about the past and the present moment but also what we intend to do in the future, including plans and goals we have. When Jane makes plans for the future, she automatically (including unconsciously) starts to look for and collect information related to her intended goals.

Imagine Jane has learned that she has an overseas business trip next month. Automatically, her behavior changes as she moves through her daily life because she knows what needs to be done: buying necessary items at the store, making reservations at the dog kennel, and making arrangements at work for her absence. Her subconscious mind will automatically bring up needed information about what she will need for the trip, and things she needs to take care of will begin to occur to her. She will change her behavior based on this important future event because she has intentionally and consciously overlaid that longer-term plan on top of her short-term day-to-day routines, which start to be adjusted to fit the new information. Jane will actually be changing the context of her relevant memories, and some of her associated day-to-day activities will have a new context.

When we make plans and manage what is going to happen in the future, it makes the future *and* present more predictable, stable, reliable, and calm—all of which are helpful for a long and healthy life, as we saw earlier. Managing the future by making plans uses our intellectual capabilities to direct our lives to unfold in efficient and predictable ways, lowering stress on a more permanent basis than simply taking time out to calm down as stress arises, which, of course, is also helpful.

Of course, plans and intentions are only as helpful as the information used to make them and the individual's ability to actualize them. It doesn't make sense to plan elaborate trips overseas, such as how to get there and where to stay, when one doesn't have a job or other means to actualize the intention. Readers probably also know that "over-planning" or "micromanaging" every little detail can also be a problem. It's important to try to be realistic because besides wasting energy, if you commit to do something, it can be stressful and disruptive to change course later. For

Jane's health framework, making more generalized visualizations (we discuss this in the next few paragraphs) or plans can make them more realistic and useful because they encompass more possible outcomes and are therefore easier to actualize.

We have been speaking of mental aspects in this chapter, but using our intellectual abilities to plan and act effectively still depends on taking care of our core physical attributes and needs. If we are busy dealing with immediate concerns (sickness, lack of sleep, etc.), they will tend to override our long-term plans until taken care of. This is natural and not meant to be viewed negatively; as we described earlier, our inner biology works this way as well, dropping long-term concerns for short-term issues, if important. The body will use flexibility now if we keep stressing it despite future ramifications. While the ability to deal with short-term uncertainty or stress is certainly valuable, planning is still important and can be used to focus that valuable attribute. For example, a talented football team may not need to stick to a good game plan to defeat a worse team with a great plan they *do* stick to, but in any case, both teams benefit greatly from the formulation and execution of good plans.

When working on specific aspects of the body, we want to also stress that physical activity is also needed to optimally form internal memory, and that is where practice sessions come in. The physical practice is "feedback" for the intentions or formulated plan and creates memory going forward towards the actual game or upcoming intended event. However, similar to what we mentioned before, this is not a micromanaged process. Jane doesn't have to tell her muscles what to do; rather, intentional outcomes are planned, pictured, and practiced, and the body tends to follow through automatically.

Of course, even a planner like Jane can't hope to plan every little detail of her future, nor is it necessary. But in the same way as her travel plans tend to change her current mental and physical behavior automatically, she can use visualizations to plan her future. In visualizing important events about her future health, for example, her subconscious mind and body will begin to plan to fit itself to that visualization, or what we call a "virtual environment" or blueprint. Especially with physical input, her body will rise to meet the (virtual) environmental demand she has created in the same way a sports psychologist trains a golfer to hit the perfect (visualized) golf shot.[32]

Virtual Environments

Jane's perception is the interface between her environment and her internal systems and memories, therefore she has another very important aspect as it pertains to health and fitness. Jane, as a human being, has the ability to "hold things in mind" (like an image), which may be somewhat separate from the actual physical environment she is in at any given time.

While we call this the ability to create a "virtual environment," we're not talking about a new technological invention or a talent. We prefer this verbiage over words like "imagination" because of the known importance of the environment in inducing changes in one's biology. This means that the environment our bodies change to fit within includes things that we hold in mind, or visualize, which is also involved—although perhaps unconsciously—when we make plans, as previously discussed. Jane can do much more than simply clear her mind to resolve stress. By training her internal systems and updating old memories, especially with long timeline visualizations, her stress levels will drop in real time, making her actually able to handle what stress does arise more easily.

When we say virtual environments can be "somewhat separate" from the actual physical environment at a given time, we don't mean to imply that the memories used to create them don't ultimately come from a past experience in an actual physical environment. Rather, our human processing power can use parts of various memories to create experiences (virtual environments) in the present moment.

A given scenario held in mind can also involve processing many different memories extrapolated into potential outcomes that have not actually been experienced yet. We don't believe is this is some magical ability; at some point in evolution, enough memory or information could be held and compared to result in this ability. Clearly, processing more information has been advantageous and, therefore, a natural outcome during evolution.

So, while we can urge Jane to make certain physical alterations to her environment, such as to solidify healthy physical surroundings, regular eating and sleeping patterns, or manage her workload and other aspects of her life when possible, Jane can also use her ability to visualize. She can create virtual environments (visualize) periodically during the day to induce positive changes to her own memory, behavior, and body going forward. As humans, we also passively create our own virtual environments automatically on a regular basis, which induce our bodies to make changes. We want Jane to begin to use this ability intentionally to manage her life in positive ways.

Virtual environments cause internal change. A simple example of this is the fact that imagining something scary brings on the simple fight-or-flight response, or certain foods bring digestive responses. In a way, Jane's body thinks what she visualizes is real. We won't go as far as discussing the details, descriptions, or theory of mental attributes, fantasies, or imagination, as this is beyond the point of this book. However, we do want to capitalize on this relationship between the mind and body. Jane can use this ability to trigger specific changes in her body as well as train her internal life over time. She can intentionally use virtual environments to affect outcomes having to do with her own body and health, rather than leaving this up to the physical environment around her. Therefore, when formulating visualizations, we could say we are making plans, or "blueprints," for our bodies to follow.

There is a long history throughout the world of using visualizations or other mental activities to affect the body—religions, meditation traditions, yoga, mental exercises, sports psychology, and more. We are not claiming anything new or special about what we are calling a "virtual environment." Rather, we believe that this is a vastly underutilized and underappreciated ability that can be a powerful tool for our own health and fitness. Indeed, many prominent medical and educational institutions now have departments dedicated to "mind-body medicine," which includes yoga, qi-gong, and other techniques to reduce stress and fight disease. We believe this field is in its infancy and that our book can help us understand *why* these techniques work and how they can be further developed to increase their use for program development going forward.

By utilizing current understandings of the evolution of the human body and related communication, we can go much further than is presented here. Further, using even the basic idea of the theory of intended evolution could change many aspects of how physiology is viewed.

How Jane lives her life—but also how she pictures and plans to live it—affects Jane's health and healthspan. With virtual environments as a management tool, Jane can begin to blueprint her future and build her framework intentionally rather than simply let her day-to-day environment and activities be the only input.

We talked about how Jane's physical activities shape her body because internal systems are intelligent. Jane's muscles adjusted and changed size when she started doing fitness classes, and then again when she quit. When repeated often enough, her body assumes an activity is the routine going forward and makes needed changes for that future. For a commonly used example of how what Jane mentally does also affects her body and internal memories, we note how sports psychologists know that *visualizing* perfect outcomes ahead of time can increase accuracy of actual outcomes in the future.[33] This is a simple example of virtual environments, and such techniques make perfect sense with the intended evolution concept: an image is visualized, which is translated inward as part of how local cells and systems perceive they will need to perform in the future. For example, with repetition and visualizing before each golf shot—followed by rounds of physical feedback—the internal memory is updated, and related changes are made.

When possible, visualizing *and* physical activity is generally much more effective than visualization alone.[34] When both the mind and the body are integrated for a given activity, all Jane's internal systems are also in alignment with her central awareness and create the most effective situation. Maximum awareness of feedback from physical activity also accelerates the learning process at all levels, meaning that paying attention to her body's feedback rather than watching TV during the physical activity (for example) is very beneficial. Therefore, when creating a virtual environment for fitness or sports, it should often include or be in conjunction with physical forms, or activities, and vice-versa.

As we mentioned earlier, Jane's minute-to-minute behavior will tend to automatically line up with a given future plans or virtual environments (visualizations): there is *cumulative progress* towards that goal. And if we monitor our thought patterns closely, when we *intend* to do something in the future, there is often already a visual component or picture there naturally. Picturing our intentions with the virtual environments of our choice is basically managing and focusing this phenomenon by adding detail and taking more time, which directs our memory and filters future incoming information in the direction of our intentions.

This said, like the need for physical action in conjunction with visualizations to get the best results in sports, it's ultimately Jane's actual behavior that gives feedback and solidifies change toward future intended goals. She will need to follow through with visualizations by way of physical activity. Therefore, she needs to also choose the real-time behaviors that begin to occur to her to augment her *cumulative directional progress*—she must make changes as she becomes aware of them. The good news is that the virtual portion of her program helps make these changes much easier than attempting change by fighting habits only as they arise. Her changes will become smoother and more natural as she trains her body and mind ahead of time.

Before moving on, we want to take a moment to look back at the two longevity strategies discussed at the end of the last chapter. The first strategy is to have as regular, calm, simple, lives of *little change*, such as those reported about in longevity villages or certain animals (lobsters or tortoises, for example). We want Jane to use this strategy for activities that most affect her core systems, those that didn't evolve to be challenged.

The second is to employ our flexibility or change potential for the goal of planning a long life. This second strategy should make more sense now in the context of virtual environments because, as humans, our main source of flexibility in dealing with change is our mental capabilities. Jane's modern environment demands many things from her that require physical flexibility for short-term troubles that pop up in our modern lifestyle, but with her powerful intellectual capacity, she can manage where and when she uses it. Jane doesn't actually have to move to a fishing village; she can create virtual environments that have some of those attributes to signal her body to use her flex potential for a long, healthy life versus short-term change.

Updating Memory

Any change, from increasing or decreasing her muscle mass to changing a habit entails some form of memory change in Jane's body. One valuable and surprising aspect of this process is due to one of the topics we discussed earlier, that Jane's mind and body aren't really separate. Rather, her mind arises out of her body, and information can move both inward from her perceptions *and* from inside up to her awareness.

Therefore, while Jane's internal systems give her relevant information from memory, they also update that memory to reflect what Jane perceives and does. They will begin to adjust and "tune" to a new environment, including virtual. Over time, they will send *different signals* back to Jane as her memory is updated. Essentially, the timelines in Jane's memory are rearranged and updated, including those affecting current behavior, old habits, and forming new ones.

Over time, Jane's mental framework automatically changes; whatever Jane does, including in her visualizations, results in new behaviors and dropping old ones that don't fit into the (new) environment she has created. *Jane is changing her sense of self.*[35]

With this proactive approach, Jane proceeds by intending change, on purpose and ahead of time, rather than just when she occasionally runs into challenges calling for change. Over time, this results in the activities and habits that don't fit into her new environment falling away naturally.

We want to reiterate that this process takes time, and our programs are not quick fixes to health or weight loss; rather, they are of a more permanent nature. Adjusting or updating memories with virtual environments entails the biology described in Chapter 1 when discussing the theory of intended evolution: Jane's systems do not simply adjust themselves based on casual short-term encounters; they wait until they are sure that the new environment is what is expected going forward. In other words, time and repetition—or, we could say, regular patterns of behavior—are needed. Random occurrences typically aren't something living cells and systems can utilize, but regular and reliable patterns that are useful are saved to memory. This also means that these types of changes are much more likely to be long-lasting and become a new way of life.

Visualizations

Included in the overall aspect of time, there are many possible inputs in our memories: sight, sound, smell, touch, and taste, for example. Therefore, anytime Jane visualizes, it is good for her to try to engage other senses while doing so because experiences are stored in the memory based on multiple sensory inputs as well. For example, if Jane is visualizing a scene with pine trees, she can try to smell them and hear the wind blowing through them in addition to picturing the image of the trees. This is similar to why physical activity augments visualization: more memory modes of input tend to create more powerful memory updates, which is a basic goal in this scenario.

We want to make clear that we are not implying anyone can change *any* behavior with virtual environments. This is an individualized process, and every person will have differing mental and memory attributes and goals and will create differing frameworks. Furthermore, many types of habits are very difficult to change and may be best left to appropriate professionals. That said, the very nature of creating one's own blueprint adds meaning, value, and also the flexibility of individualization for almost anyone to utilize.

Mind-Body Fitness and Medicine

In today's modern society, it is not surprising that much of what is being called "mind-body medicine" or "mind-body fitness" focuses on practices or techniques that have been shown to be effective in reducing stress. We believe that the understanding presented here can help not only Jane, but also yoga teachers, fitness trainers, healthcare companies and institutions, or others to expand on these current ideas and develop new techniques and programs to better their clients' lives. It is time for the role of our mental abilities in affecting our health to be taken seriously and for us to begin to use our individual and innate *internal medicine* as the basis for our own personalized health and fitness.

While studying the effects of stress has historically been instrumental in the West in showing the link between mental states and health, we believe mind-body fitness and medicine can widen its paradigm well beyond current techniques, although these are clearly valuable.[36] Indeed, we see a proliferation of mind-body medicine programs, research, and even classes at healthcare institutions and universities. The fact that the perceived environment induces biological change, coupled with the knowledge that we have the ability to *intentionally* create our own virtual environments through visualizations, gives us a powerful tool for our own health that is just beginning to be utilized. Spending enough time visualizing a long and healthy future, for example, leads not only to a greater likelihood of the future vision planned for but to a healthier state *now*.

Programs can be created and tailored by inventing situations needed to induce internal activity that supports a given function, remodels the body in a specific way, and retains important areas of flexibility and function into old age.

Furthermore, most currently used fitness activities can be included—or adjusted, if need be—for the long-term goals of a given individual. They may also be made more effective when viewed in a larger framework by adding visualizations to augment a given activity or even simply making sure one's mind is engaged in some way during that activity.

For example, when Jane goes running, she can do so with a purpose, her mind can be monitoring her body internally when possible and even visualize what is going on internally at times. In our opinion, paying attention to her running is much more effective than running while watching TV or listening to the news on her headphones. This is because being aware of her internal functions during a physical activity, for example, increases communication and reinforces the activity's importance to her local systems. Her "awareness" is in unity with—*in sync with*—the intelligence of her internal systems. When we approach a task and begin to do it, the body then provides feedback, but when watching TV while running or biking, there is a split in attention, and the feedback loop is less effective.

Walking is a very beneficial activity and uses very basic evolutionary functions. But when out for a walk, it is helpful to be engaged in walking and the surroundings as opposed to reflecting on your problems because by doing so, you're essentially reinforcing their importance and inhibiting the release of related stress. Visualizing certain functions inside your body during your walk or even a yoga class can augment the effectiveness of these activities, including as stress relief. In a more general way, we can visualize a different environment when feeling stressed, one that *counteracts* the stress. It is easy to say, "Don't think of your problems," or, "Clear your mind." However, in practice, not thinking about your problems or clearing your mind can certainly be quite difficult at times. However, visualizations can be used to stop a busy mind much more easily than trying to stop one's thoughts by "not thinking."

Another idea we like is to break up Jane's thinking activities with physical activities in which her thinking or worrying is automatically disengaged. This can happen without visualization if the body takes over our awareness and an activity is happening spontaneously. For example, going for a walk is usually not as effective at halting worry or stress as a game like ping-pong. These kinds of activities tend to automatically reduce or eliminate stressful thoughts because the mind is fully engaged in the activity. Playful and fun activities also tend to stimulate and balance the endocrine hormones and are involved in the learning process as we can see during development. We could say the chemistry of play is a learning and creativity pathway in the body.[37]

As many modern companies—including Jane's—have found, fifteen minutes of a playful activity like ping-pong every few hours to break up long days of brain work tends to be effective in reducing overall stress and boosting creativity. While some people tend to think of such activities in the workplace as frivolous passing fads or a waste of time, such ideas are actually emerging out of effectiveness and need. While it may not be known why they work, intuitively, people know that play relieves stress and makes their days go more smoothly and effectively. This is not to say that many other relaxation techniques, such as mentioned earlier, aren't helpful—including ones to clear the mind—but we believe visualizations and the Intended Evolution Fitness framework can increase the effectiveness of many current practices.

The Intended Evolution Framework

Finally, we want talk about the idea of Jane creating her Intended Evolution framework: a long-term—even lifelong—framework, or visualization for herself, which is related to the long-term planning discussed earlier. We include this framework visualization in the next chapter, so feel free to jump ahead and then come back to this section to learn more about the general concepts.

We have mentioned in general terms about the way environments (including virtual ones) change memories, patterns of thought, and behavior. We also said the nature of information (including in our memory) is a pattern, which implies a time factor.[38] Memories are related to each other and are used based on time, among other things. In other words, our memories have information patterns that cover different lengths of time (we have used the term "timelines") and are used and updated in relation to each other based on their timeframe or length. We wanted to repeat this here to emphasize the value of Jane creating a lifelong framework for herself. By creating a lifelong timeline, her memories and perceptions will begin to get their context from it, changing her sense of self, and behaviors.

For example, two very similar weather patterns will take on different meanings in the context of a longer timeline: what season it is. This is why, as we said before, we can notice that a long-term plan, especially when important and meaningful, tends to affect our thinking and behavior now: *short-term patterns get some of their meaning, or context, from longer-term ones.* This is important to Jane in that the larger (longer) the framework she creates, the more other plans, behaviors, and activities come under it and are managed by it. This is like a sports team trying to plan an entire season—or multiple seasons—which shapes all the upcoming trades for players, and even current day-to-day practices sessions.

The Intended Evolution Framework is meant to hold Jane's entire lifespan and she will be creating a *lifelong memory pattern* that all related shorter patterns will slowly re-arrange, or "shift," to fit within. This works as described earlier with Jane planning a trip to Europe in the future: short-term thinking and behaviors will change to fit the plan. With repetition, Jane can automatically begin a managed change of her everyday experiences to actualize the plans in her framework.

When she visualizes a long and healthy life over and over again, short- and medium-term factors (habits, plans, etc.) will be re-contextualized and adjusted based on the visualizations. Each short-term event or accomplished goal that is in line with her framework creates positive feedback and becomes another step that accumulates progress towards her goals and even her ultimate goal, a long happy healthspan. Her body will sense events working against it and alert Jane so she can make adjustments accordingly. As we have said, Jane's sense of self will change, which is much more powerful than reacting only when problems arise.

The idea is for Jane to create her lifelong framework based on where she has been, where she is currently, and where she wants to go. For optimal effectiveness, she should create it so it includes realistic and important goals that she really wants to see happen and with which she will follow through. Furthermore, although there is always uncertainty about many aspects of her future, she can still include very detailed things (added intensity) about her future health and looks as well as the activities she wants to be able to do.

Is There Optimal Functioning or Fitness?

Optimal functioning or fitness is no simple topic, and we realize there is no single answer; rather, it is different for each individual. However, the ideas we have presented on the topic throughout this book include a framework visualization (next chapter) to help each individual maximize his or her healthspan.

Basically, we believe each person can attempt to find an optimal line in the use of one's flexibility capacity. But people need to know their individual goals and ascertain what time frames they are talking about: where is Jane within her lifecycle or lifespan, and where does she want to go? Trying to ascertain what is "optimal" in regards to health and fitness implies a goal to be reached, whether it is to look or feel a certain way, be able to achieve certain tasks or goals, or something else entirely. Of course, there may be multiple goals, and while they may vary with each individual, they can still be part of the overall plan. We believe strongly that creating a lifelong blueprint or framework to "hang" other activities on, or "contextualize" them, is an important tool for such optimization.

Therefore, health and fitness shouldn't be viewed as simply trying to correct other things one does during the day, week, or year, but it also has to do with aligning each moment to fit longer-term goals and accumulate progress towards them. Ultimately, a major point often missed in today's fast-paced world is that what you plan to do *in the future* affects the state of your health and wellness *today*.

While each experienced moment in time is being input as the environment that affects our future, it is also our future plans that, in turn, affect each experienced present moment.

Chapter 6

JANE'S IE PROGRAM

We have discussed why Jane should manage her flex capacity intentionally to achieve her future goals as optimally as possible and that planning for these goals tends to change her choices, actions, and health today. Now, let's take a look at how she can put all the pieces together to create a lifelong timeline for herself as well as some activities for her day-to-day health and fitness. Our suggestions here for Jane are a small piece of the Fit-150 weight loss and metabolism program that Dr. Zhang invented more than ten years ago for people like Jane, and those with worse problems, such as diabetes.

The Intended Evolution Health & Fitness Framework: The Mind's "Scaffolding"

As we move through life, we essentially build another blueprint—or "framework"—on top of what we were born with. We also use our perception, intentions, and intelligence to build a knowledge base in this lifetime. For example, language is a sort of framework we learn as we grow in order to make sense of the world around us and communicate with others about it. Then, much of what we intellectually learn and use later in life is hung on this "scaffolding of language," so to speak.

There are many other factors that form our mental "framework" as we grow from family interactions or schooling or by training for a job or profession. Our experiences are then based on—but also update—the past framework of understanding, which is essentially part of our sense of self. As we move through life, the mental framework we use to make sense of it changes based on what we do, intend to do, and—more generally—our experiences. Our metal frameworks constantly shift and change as new information comes in and changes the meaning of our previously saved memories. Intentionally managing our frameworks means actively managing our lives.

As Jane intentionally builds her intended evolution framework for a very long and healthy lifespan, all the other information, having shorter timelines, will begin to gather context from the plan she builds. A lifelong framework, or "blueprint," creates a situation where shorter-term activities become related to long-term goals, making progress towards them more likely. Her behavior and thoughts will begin to "tune" to this new plan she builds, and over time, they will begin to shift to accommodate it. When Jane focuses on goals in the future, including near the end of her life when, while old, she still enjoys life and her needed functions are still working well, all her systems will begin to plan for these intentional outcomes.

Jane's Healthspan Optimization Framework Visualization

First of all, there is no need to do this visualization every day; two to three times a week is enough. This visualization encompasses her whole life and can take practice and patience. For some people, this will be easier after some practice, while others may not require it. This visualization can also be used in a stand-alone fashion (without physical exercise). We present it first because its all-encompassing nature makes it perhaps the most powerful tool where the overall healthspan is concerned.

You should start in a comfortable position, whether sitting, standing, or lying down. Take a deep breath, and relax. Relax your eyes, face, jaw, neck, shoulder, back, arms, fingers, legs, feet, and toes.

See yourself today, but in a natural setting you remember that was special and happy; positive, playful, and grateful emotions are important during the visualization both physically, as we've noted, and because they are carried into memory updates that occur. As we mentioned when discussing longevity, when building her life's framework, we want Jane to borrow the strategy from long-lived lifestyles to use stable environmental signals. She can visualize herself sitting in a natural area like an old pine forest with large trees and the sun shining, where things are very calm and relaxed. The key here is *consistency* and *predictability* of environmental signals: a pine forest, sun shining through the trees, is an ancient evolutionary signal recognized by our internal life and connects the rest of the visualization to Jane's DNA. Therefore, not only (as we noted earlier) is this is the opposite of what causes mental overload and stress, but it also helps her match this lifetime's framework, which she is building, to her DNA blueprint, augmenting memory updates.

1.) As you sit in that place, slowly go back in time, seeing yourself getting younger and younger. You can skip several years to start, and then use fewer gaps at a younger age. Here is a suggestion for Jane:

50 ⇨ 40 ⇨ 33 ⇨ 28 ⇨ 23 ⇨ 18 ⇨ 13 ⇨
10 ⇨ 7 ⇨ 5 ⇨ 4 ⇨ 3 ⇨ 2 ⇨ 1 ⇨

Go all the way back to when you were born—you are in your mother's arms, everything is perfect, and all your needs are taken care of.

You can spend a bit more time at the young ages and as a newborn. This first part is basically a review of your life up to this point.

2.) Then, slowly go back up to your current age, seeing yourself growing, and then go beyond:

6 months ⇨ 1 ⇨ 2 ⇨ 3 ⇨ 4 ⇨ 5 ⇨
10 ⇨ 15 ⇨ 20 ⇨ 25 ⇨ 30 ⇨40 ⇨
50 ⇨ 60 ⇨ 70 ⇨ 80 ⇨ 90 ⇨ 100 ⇨
110 ⇨ 120 ⇨ 140 ⇨ 160

Imagine being very healthy and happy as you go: healthy joints, teeth, and vision at all ages you visit. Here, you are rewriting your life, building the Intended Evolution Framework for a long, healthy, and happy life. For the things that have already happened, you can highlight the things that fit in well with a long healthspan and the goals you decide to put in your framework for the future. For the part that has not happened yet, you want to choose some general but important events and put them out on your future timeline, things you really want to see and do in the future. For example, you remain very healthy and perhaps are still enjoying a sport you like at an old age, or you are seeing great-grandchildren and even *their* children playing around you. When you reach the maximum age you have chosen, your longest goal in life, sit there for a few moments and see yourself still fully functional as an old but not decrepit person and "remember" all the things that have happened during the life you created in a positive and grateful manner.

3.) Then, start the journey back down in age: 160 ⇨ 140 ⇨ . . . back to a newborn state. In this step, you are reviewing the life you have created. Spend some extra time on important events and goals and then again in your younger years. Younger years are times of great flexibility, and your body can benefit greatly from revisiting these ages. Visualizing back to your young ages also gives context to the future part of your journey; the things that have already happened point to *why* you are where you are now and also where you are going. This also personalizes the whole process, our early lives help make sense of everything: where we are now, and where we are going.

4.) Finally, turn around again and progress back to the age you are now. This time, it is more reaffirming. Think, *Yes, this has happened, it led to today, and so the rest will happen, too. All done!*

Commentary

First, when you go through the healthspan years you have chosen, it is with positive, grateful emotions, which help balance the hormones and are healthy in nature. By visualizing your entire healthspan, you are saving this very long timeline to memory, which will update everything else in your framework over time, including today's behavior and all your memories. Over time, you are re-contextualizing where you are headed, where you are now, and the memories of where you have been—essentially, your very sense of self.

Therefore, regardless of your past, you will see it in a good light over time, getting you to where you are right now. The future years are also positive and fulfilling, and you set general "landmarks" and images. By "landmarks," we mean for you to picture yourself doing things you really want to do in the future or events you really want to see. Although general in nature (you might see yourself very healthy playing your favorite sport at one hundred years old), *you see the pictures in detail.* As you progress to what most people think is very old and near death (say, one hundred or one hundred twenty), you look much younger and can still do all the things you want and can clearly go further, even if you decide to stop there.

At Jane's visualized age of eighty, she will only be middle-aged, maybe with only a few grey hairs, and will still be able to do nearly whatever she wants. Of course, you may not be sure about many things, and you want to be realistic, but you only need a few ideas to start, and keeping them general means they won't become outdated. You can also add new things over time or update previous ones.

Why 150 or 160?

People have differing ideas as to how long the human lifespan can be, and of course, it is probably different for each person. Here, we are using the second longevity strategy: directing our flex potential towards the demand for a long life. We are challenging the normal lifespan so the body will respond by using its resources in a way that stretches out the amount of functional time it needs to last. We know people can live well past one hundred, and stretching our healthspan timeline to 150 or 160 simply challenges the body to try to realize this goal, creating changes now to meet it, which leads to healthier choices, actions, and health today.

However, it is important to choose an age you can believe in but also view as realistic. Visualizing an unrealistic framework that doesn't match our DNA, such as demanding something like immortality, is a waste of time and energy. Also, many people will say they don't want to live to be that old because they picture themselves as decrepit, or they might simply believe that if they do live that long, all their friends will be gone, making the idea seem strange or sad to them. It is fine to choose a younger age, but it is also important to know that by planning for a very long life, the body automatically starts planning for it now, meaning you can become healthier now, which, of course, is a fine goal.

Weight Loss

Jane's short-, medium-, and long-term goals were to burn calories, lose weight, and be healthy. As we have said, we don't think that burning maximum calories is always in line with weight loss or long-term health goals, so our recommendations will start with weight loss. We have discovered quite simple ways to create demands on the body that induce fat reduction directly. We find our unique techniques more effective than trying to use large muscles to burn fat because our techniques signal the body that the primary goal is to use the fat resulting in taking in *fewer* calories, not more.

The activities below (which can be seen on video at www.intendedevolution.com) signal the body to remove fat because it is a hindrance given the new activities the body is experiencing. To remove the fat, the body will use it for fuel rather than reenergizing entirely through consuming more calories. What we call "The Shake" or "The Twist," combined with visualizations, tells the body that extra fat is in the way in those areas and needs to be removed, resulting in a naturally reduced appetite as the body removes it by using it for fuel as opposed to new food intake. Like muscle or bone remodeling, we have discovered that fat can also be remodeled based on where the internal systems sense shaking and movement. We believe this fat can even be associated with the internal organs, although we have not done a study on this. These activities naturally reduce the appetite rather than forcing the body to endure the torture of trying to eat less through willpower, which normally can be very difficult, especially during high calorie burn and muscle-building activities. These examples of physical activities are directly in line with Jane's weight loss and long-term health goals, as well as how her internal systems work and evolved (see *Weight-loss Theory* later in this chapter).

The Shake

The goal here is simply to stimulate or shake the fat tissue in the body. The simplest shake activity can be done standing with legs shoulder-width apart and flexing the feet and ankles: coming up off the heels and then back down on them quickly so as to feel the fat (mostly in the abdomen and torso here) moving up and down (Jane will want to wear her sports bra). The idea is a vigorous movement in order to get the sensation of maximum tissue (skin and fat) movement. When the body senses the repeated movement or shaking, it will automatically know things have changed: given this new activity, a new body type is needed.

Furthermore, by using only the smaller (lower leg and foot) muscles, the body is not signaled to build much muscle (as when the large upper leg muscles are worked) and, therefore, won't need to take in calories from protein to build them up. There are many possible versions of this; we are using this simple example for the purpose of understanding how a physical example would fit the theory. Another simple example could be jogging in place or advancing an inch or so at a time, forward backward, and side to side, again primarily flexing the ankles and feet—a "stutter step," so to speak. A side-to-side stutter step can be added to shake the fat sideways and stimulate it in a different but similar way, adding to the signal that the fat there is a problem. Fitness or yoga trainers and teachers can invent many versions of this type of action to maximize shaking with minimal muscle use.

Visualizations for The Shake

- First of all, we want to say that having the mind engaged is very important because it helps send the message to eliminate fat and updates that memory in the tissues. Standing on a vibrating platform watching TV or reading is not nearly as effective as actively being involved in the shaking activity.

- Before starting her shaking, Jane should sit relaxed for a minute or two and picture herself the way she would like to look, perhaps as she looked when younger or maybe using the model of another person whose body she thinks she should look like. A realistic projection of herself in the future communicates to her bodies systems that this is where they are headed.

- Then, as she shakes, Jane can visualize her fat shaking and beginning to melt away or perhaps that she is her younger self with the extra fat shaking and disappearing. This can be individualized, since people will be drawn to different ideas on these motifs. As long as the visualizations make sense, can be realistically believed, and fat is visualized to be melting away, they can do the job.

- The important physical part is to create activities that require quick movements—any activity where the fat can be felt to be shaking, such as very short steps or hops that allow the benefit of feeling tissue movement without undue stress on joints. Again, the more individualized, the more sense it makes and the more believable for each individual. Students and teachers can share ideas on how to get the feeling of more tissue shaking and create their own forms.

- Jane can start with whatever is comfortable but hopefully work up to twenty to thirty minutes three times per week. She can incorporate many techniques as long as they entail shaking of the tissues and can also put some twisting in the workout.

The Twist

This activity stimulates the fat specifically around the middle and targets fat loss in that area. With arms out to the side you rotate your upper body to the left and look behind you as far as is comfortable while your lower body moves to the right (standing on the right leg your left knee comes up and moves across the body to the right). Then, repeat in the opposite direction. This signals the body that the twisting fat is in the way of this new activity and needs to be removed. You can take small steps forward to help keep balanced as you go back and forth. Do this eighteen times each way.

Visualizations for the Twist

- Again, Jane should sit relaxed for a couple of minutes and picture herself the way she would like to look—her future body image—which sets the goal for her body.

- As she twists from side to side, Jane should visualize her twisting motions as squeezing liquid fat out, like wringing out a wet towel. She can also hold the idea in mind that there will always be plenty of food in the future and there is no need to keep it stored.

- With one twist meaning one to the left and one to the right, Jane can do eighteen repetitions once or twice during her shaking time. This is very quick and simple and can be done at other times during the day when she gets a chance also.

Twist & Shake Comments

- These activities and related visualizations make the body aware of extra tissue that needs to be removed wherever it shakes.

- Notice the goal of only using small muscles when shaking, since a lot of tissue movement can result by flexing only the ankles. Because large muscles aren't used much, there is no signal to eat more to fuel muscle growth. We have found that shaking and twisting results in loss of appetite over time as the body begins to use the fat and suppresses the appetite. There is active stimulation of fat tissue without the caloric burn of using large muscles, resulting in fat remodeling where it was shaken or twisted.

- These can both usually be done even by very overweight people as long as they can flex their ankles. It can also be done almost anywhere, and five minutes here and there along with the visual of fat melting is highly beneficial and reinforces the message to remove fat.

- Shaking, twisting, and other fat stimulating activities can be formulated to be much less stressful on joints and other parts of the body than running or many other activities. We have developed many other forms but the point here is more to interest the reader in the concepts and theory of how to induce the body to drop fat and reduce the appetite in the process.

- Finally, like activities such as running, shaking augments fluid metabolism and movement of lymph, and those areas can be especially targeted if needed.

- If you need help understanding what these movements look like, you can view a helpful video of these forms at www.intendedevolution.com.

Weight-Loss Theory

The above is a portion of a weight-loss program we have developed, and while we have not done a scientific study, we have seen remarkable results so far.

When viewed with our framework in mind, we believe that distance running can be seen as a "proof of concept" for the shake and twist. Distance running is well-known to induce weight loss and results in a "runner's body," so to speak. While all weight loss ultimately comes from using more calories than taken in, and running certainly burns calories, it is unique compared to many other high-burn workout programs. We believe that runners drop mass, including fat and especially in the (relatively unused) upper body, because the body is *responding* to the constant shaking and pounding. The body will shed the weight because the body "knows" that the movements and demands of running mean that weight is a hindrance to this activity.

Finally, the body's fat is recently being viewed as an endocrine organ and affects the entire endocrine system,[39] including the hormones that control nutritional intake. Through testing Jane's recommendations, we have found this makes sense in that directly stimulating fat by twisting and shaking can kick-start endocrine activity, balancing hormones and lifting one's mood—even relatively quickly in sedentary people. Jane will notice more energy and less stress well before she actually starts losing weight. Essentially, we have found that like other physical activities induce the body to add or take away tissue (muscle or bone remodeling), this is also the case with adipose tissue. In this case, stimulation as described here signals the body to reduce it in a given area.

Because it takes time and repetition for the body to consider the activity as the "new normal," this program can take longer than crash courses, quick-loss diets, or weight-loss pills. However, we have found that because the entire endocrine system is engaged and appetite is lowered, it is much easier to keep the weight off. Furthermore, these activities and seeing oneself looking a certain way in the visualizations are updating memory in the body over time and slowly changing one's sense of self.

Eyes

The importance of vision in our lives cannot be emphasized enough. Visual information dominates our senses, and light is such a large part of the environment that most complex lifeforms have some sort of light-sensing capabilities. From insects to fish, from fish to man, vision plays an important role in survival and is a very evolutionarily core function. However, environmental changes and specialization in our modern society have weakened our visual abilities because we live in relative safety and no longer rely on our acute vision to hunt and avoid predators. Today, we also don't require the same amount of movement of the eyes as we did in the past. Due to these functional changes (looking at computers rather than searching for food or danger), we are more likely to develop degenerative diseases such as macular degeneration. Furthermore, by requiring excessive and constant focus, using artificial light, and specializing in reading, watching TV, and using computers, our eyes can be constantly fatigued, leading to near-sightedness or other troubles. Vision exercises help relax and rest the eyes and promote more circulation and movement in all parts of the eyes. They put a functional demand on the eyes but do not stress them.

The Eye Roll

This is essentially a very simple eye exercise that brings fluid and resources into the eyes. Get in a comfortable position with your head straight. Try to look at the top of your head; you may feel a slight strain as you try to look higher. Roll your eyes to the right, and try to see your right ear. Then, continue downward to see your chin. Finally, continue to roll your eyes and see your left ear. Finish at the starting position to complete round one.

Do three rounds in one direction and then three rounds rolling in the other direction. You can visualize expanding your eye sockets as you look around. Removal of contacts is recommended. Stop if your eyes feel any major discomfort.

Notes on the Eyes

Today, the need for better visual performance is, frankly, optional since our vision demands don't match their evolutionary use. A main problem comes from the lack of circulation around and to the eye. We may not be able to revert to our old ways, but we can prevent potential problems by providing mental and physical challenges to increase the functional demand upon our eyes. This exercise provides both because it increases the range of motion and challenges the mechanisms of the eyes. It forces the eyes to look where they cannot and allows the eyes to use their full range of motion.

By pushing this movement to the limits—to where it is very rarely used—we can require the eyes to do more than today's limited functions, like watching a screen right in front of us. This also strengthens the muscle around the eye and increases circulation locally. This is an exercise that can be done very quickly and anywhere at any time. This exercise can have tremendous positive effects on macular degeneration, especially if started early enough.

Teeth

Although great strides have been made in modern corrective dentistry, keeping healthy teeth is still the best option and is very important because healthy teeth are an important part of the health of the whole body. Due to the quality and form of food we consume, we no longer have to use our teeth in the ways we evolved to. For example, processed foods give our teeth less of a challenge than the diets we evolved to eat. Use of our jaw and related muscles too far below normal historical (evolutionarily) norms may also affect other related functions in areas such as the nose or digestion. As the first part of our digestion, the jaw and teeth are part of a core system that we don't want to allow to degrade. Furthermore, when the teeth start to have trouble, it is something to pay attention to, not just because the teeth are important but as a sign that overall health is declining.

Maintaining good dental health from the intended evolution fitness perspective means pressing the urgency and usefulness of the teeth and jaw in terms of their original functions. Challenging the function of the teeth and jaw to make them stronger reminds the body that they are still very much needed and affects all related systems, keeping them strong as well.

Of course, we also don't want to further wear out the teeth and jaw through overuse. Here are a couple of simple forms that use the mind to demand challenging tasks for the teeth and jaw.

Tapping

Tapping your teeth together is basically a challenge to your teeth and jaw and signals the body keep this function strong, not unlike using muscles will make them stronger. With today's diet of soft food, we need to create challenges to signal the teeth to stay strong and not only react to the modern diet.

Visualizations for Tapping

First, we prepare the teeth and jaw area to be strong by making a small framework or visualization for the area. Doing this can enhance the result of ensuing physical challenges:

- First, know that healthy teeth are a part a long and healthy life, and quickly picture yourself with great teeth for your entire healthspan.
- Picture your teeth like little containers (for example, plastic bags) filled up with bright white light. Picture the bones of the mouth also full of light.
- At the end of the visualization, you should feel like you want to do something with your teeth, like you want some physical challenge.

- Now, take a deep breath and visualize you are tapping through a piece of cardboard or thin piece of wooden board with your teeth. Because the board is made of wood or tough paper, it has some elasticity. So, if your motion is not crisp and quick, you will not be able to tap through the board. Do this positively, and see yourself getting through.

Now, actually tap your teeth together—but not *too* vigorously; you don't want to damage your teeth. After a while, you'll find a comfortable zone. If done correctly, you may feel like you really want to bite on something or tap through something.

Notes on Teeth

Besides doing this routine a couple times a week, Jane should also take this into her real life and really pay attention while she is eating. She can even make up her own visualization about digesting her food. This is obviously not something for meals that often entail discussion and social situations, but there are usually plenty of times when Jane can really pay attention to her eating and utilize what she learned here.

How Can We Best Optimize Our Virtual Environment Capacity?

This applies to the above discussion of the intended evolution framework visualization but also to all the visualizations presented, including what the reader may do from other mind-body practices. Basically, the points below can be summed up as factors that augment, or are present, when one truly intends to get something done or reach a goal. Whereas natural selection has to do only with challenges from the environment affecting survival, intended evolution has to do with the internal drive to intentionally manage the direction one goes and choosing which challenges to engage and how.

- **Time and Repetition:** both are needed to update our internal memories. Changes or updates are not made until a cell or system perceives that the current situation is likely to persist. In general, life adjusts itself to beneficial patterns as opposed to occurrences not thought to repeat in the future.

- **Need or Importance:** Of course, these are interrelated, and something very important to us (or needed by us or a system) will tend to update memory more quickly. An example we don't want to use here is a traumatic event, which can, for example, update previous memory after only that single event.

- **Intensity and Detail:** Related to the above, this helps "convince" the body. When visualizing certain scenarios, paying close attention and creating detail is important because it makes it more real and more intense, as well as more important.

- **Fun or Enjoyment:** Basically, curiosity, fun, playfulness, and enjoyment are mindsets of the natural learning mode and unleash intentional drive. We can see it in children: these positive states are associated with our natural pathways to change. This is an aspect that can and should be taken into consideration in many areas of people's lives and activities, including their health and fitness regimes. A miserable experience is the opposite of this and will tend to be counterproductive as well as difficult to follow up with.

- **Energy:** We call energy the currency of change, and using it efficiently is important for a long healthspan. This has to be taken into account in health and fitness because we are talking about making changes to everything from our physical bodies to habits and lifestyles. Everyone has differing amounts of energy to put into a health and fitness program, and it is very important to work within a person's ability regarding the needed effort of given activities.

Otherwise, the plan will be miserable and hard to continue regularly.

Summation

Jane can pick and choose which forms to do when it is convenient to do for her. Some parts of her program clearly need special time out and privacy, but some can be done at any time, including periodically during the day. This is important because it is creating regular patterns of behavior, and regularity is important in inducing the body to make changes. She can also use the principles spelled out in her program in various other activities in her everyday life. We want to also reiterate that it is very important to utilize the points above about augmenting the *intention* to actualize the visualization and goals.

Change is an active, intentional process, and although there are many programs and activities available in the fitness realm that can augment Jane's goals and fit her framework, she should choose those that she enjoys and will really intend to continue in the future.

Day-to-Day Examples of Jane's Plan

We feel it is very important that health and fitness needs to be a part of our day-to-day activities and fit our lifestyles to be truly adhered to and, therefore, provide long-term benefit. Our suggestions for Jane can be easily implemented, as well as adjusted over time for changes of her normal daily routine, allowing for long-term results without worrying about missing one of her current workouts or yoga classes.

At the start of a usual Monday, Jane would wake up like any other day and can now begin to take thirty seconds to gather her thoughts and glance ahead to what her day holds. She forms a very general timeline for the day, such as breakfast, work, lunch with a co-worker, work, make and eat dinner, and finally, some relaxing time before bed.

She then gets up and does some yoga stretching, which is something she does every morning, and with our methods she would incorporate more mental imaging of the insides of her body becoming extra flexible, even more than she is now. She can also picture a "role model" before she starts, someone who is very flexible to try to emulate, or certain animals, like a snake, which parts of her body can become more like. As with any activity, there is also an acknowledgement that this helps create progress to her long personal timeline she has created for herself. Perhaps she can visualize being very flexible at a very old age . . . She can also briefly remember when she was younger and could do remarkable flexibility activities.

After her shower and while getting ready for work, Jane can do a couple of minutes of eye exercise to start the day off sharp and clear. During breakfast, Jane pays extra attention and fully enjoys of all the aspects of her food—the looks, smell, and taste. Then, after breakfast and brushing her teeth, she inserts a minute of teeth tapping with the related visualizations in the same way, seeing very healthy teeth for her long life.

While getting dressed, Jane can take a moment to put herself in the right frame of mind for the upcoming work day, looking forward to the upcoming challenges and highlights as well as the unexpected and new.

All of this added activity has probably taken five minutes or less to Jane's previous morning routine, and during the day, she takes small breaks and finds a spot where she can do a little twisting or shaking when she feels fatigued. This signals the body to use the fat as well as gets her fluid metabolism moving again if she has been sitting for periods of time.

During lunch, Jane has a great meeting with a friend and can take a moment afterwards to be grateful that this and other parts of her morning have fit in well with her long personal timeline, helping create cumulative progress towards her future goals. Everything positive and enjoyable should be acknowledged and used to fuel her overall healthspan framework.

On the way home from work, she hears an interesting and thought-provoking podcast and makes a mental note that being able to learn new and interesting ideas is something she would like to do throughout her healthspan and as long as possible. She may decide to add a related goal in her visualization for the timeline of her overall Framework next time she adjusts it.

Jane decides to try a new recipe for dinner that evening, something extra healthy and delicious she found online, and she is grateful she decided to eat healthy that night and pictures her body benefiting from that decision. Proper nutrition for her body is part of her plan for maximum healthspan and so results in her enjoying it as well as the positive things during that day even more.

Since it is an off-day in terms of exercise for Jane, she does a few minutes of shaking that evening and she does a short version of her personalized healthspan framework visualization before bed and perhaps briefly updating it, incorporating briefly new things that fit in and perhaps eliminating some things that don't.

For this typical day, the suggested elements add perhaps fifteen minutes in total, but over time it will change the mental framework of a lot of her activities, giving them a more cohesive meaning in terms of her overall lifespan framework.

The next day is Tuesday, one of the two days a week Jane goes out jogging. Nothing changes from Monday's routine, but now she augments her run by fitting it into the context of her overall framework, seeing that this will help her keep her mobile for her entire healthspan, and she adds some mental imaging as well. She can visualize an admired runner with the body she is looking for, for example, or go with an evolutionary scenario likely in her DNA such as chasing prey, a gazelle escaping a predator, or a combination. There are many personalized scenarios that Jane could come up with, and others can come up with different versions. The key here is that every step and movement can be filled with purpose, creating important demands for the body to respond to. Even sensory functions, such as vision or hearing, can be used in a given scenario to sharpen their functioning. In particular, trying to see detailed distant things is something that is very valuable because nearly all of our modern-day demands on vision are close-up and have limited context, like things on paper or a computer screen. Every time Jane runs and even with every step she takes, having purpose will accumulate progress towards shaping her body's form and function to match her overall plan or framework she has created.

Wednesday is one of the two days of the week Jane goes to the gym, where she has set goals with the help of her fitness trainer, who also tracks and monitors her progress. The framework visualization and techniques don't interfere with her activities there; rather, they augment them, and her gym activities can fit into her overall healthspan optimization framework.

An example of augmenting her gym activities could be focusing internally on her cardiovascular system during activities, which are conducive to doing so. This is something Jane wants to make sure to focus on because cardiovascular disease runs in her family. Various internal visualizations targeting blood vessel elasticity and muscle activity after her workout is complete is very useful and takes just a few minutes. She can also insert this goal of cardiovascular health as a focal point into her healthspan framework, setting related goals and events way out on her timeline. Many of the changes occur by way of refocusing of certain aspects of her activities to move forward toward her healthspan goals, also meaning Jane will tend to gravitate towards activities that augment her overall healthspan framework.

It's now the end of the week, and Jane will do a full healthspan optimization visualization, which is now quite familiar to her as she constructed it and has been updating it slowly for a few months now. The past portion of the timeline is now fairly stable and fixed, although new information may emerge as some alterations to memory occur over time. But with every week, new experiences, likes or dislikes, and new goals and interests all need to be accounted for by updating the overall timeline. Jane has chosen the end of each week to upload the newest version of her framework to use in her visualization. This continuous purposeful updating and repeating the visualization a couple of times a week give the body a meaningful demand for change.

The weekend starts with Jane's normal suggested activities described earlier, but the day turns stressful quickly with a minor car accident and the news that someone close to her was diagnosed with a serious disease. Life can throw a lot at us, and sometimes feeling down is the most natural reaction. It is not unhealthy to feel sad, angry, or agitated, but many emotions—even "good ones" such as joy and excitement—can wear us out if persistent and left unchecked.

A major benefit of Jane visualizing her long-term timeline is that it puts Jane's short-term situations into a much larger context. Jane's many internal systems, which are involved in her emotional responses, are working together and help balance each other to meet the larger goal. By focusing on the big picture a few times a week, short-term events, including emotional swings, are softened and not as dramatic, providing much needed stability, even when things get messy.

The healthspan visualization is meant to "blueprint" personal and positive life experiences as foundations Jane uses to manage her drive and direct it towards a maximum healthspan. She will tend to seek out experiences that are similar in nature to the framework she is building towards her long-term goals. The consistency of the framework she's creating provides a stable mental and physical comfort zone for Jane when things are tough and unexpected events bring high emotions.

Of course, blowing off steam with exercise routines during such times when possible is also beneficial in the short-term, but maintaining a larger view tends to automatically balance emotional events quicker and more easily while also using other solutions.

Chapter 7

CONCLUSION

Applying the concepts of intended evolution to health, fitness, and mind-body medicine is simply a new way of organizing several well-established ideas about how our bodies function into a system that focuses on an individual's health. It is well known that our physical bodies and our mental processes are one functioning unit, and the brain's importance to the body's survival is no less than the lungs or the heart. But the human mind offers us a special evolutionary advantage in the ability to reason out results, anticipate what is expected to come in the future, and apply them to our physiologies.

Essentially, humans can plan or forecast scenarios that have not taken place or even things that are merely possibilities. By making intelligent projections and choices for action regarding that expected future, the body will begin to change itself *now* to actualize those scenarios. Therefore, the brain's role involves interpretation of sensory input, leading to the body's response: our mental processes can lead to change in body chemistry, such as hormones, which in turn produces larger, more systematic physical responses.

We also know that our minds and bodies are keenly attuned to evolutionary factors, such as survival chances, environmental signals, and social mating advantages. Our concepts simply take advantage of this and the human intelligence factor to focus on health.

There are already a lot of well-practiced activities that use these capabilities in more limited situations and in other areas. There are endless examples of people using their intelligence and planning capabilities in everyday life to actualize their future intentions. These are actually very advanced evolutionary functions. Other examples are more direct, forecasting future scenarios such as stock market and other investment plans. Sports psychology is another area directly related to affecting our own bodies and its memories by using our advanced human mental functions.

Yet, there is no system which—instead of just focusing on specific tasks, such as to run faster, jump higher, or make a given shot—focuses directly on the overall human physical condition and its "fitness" in regard to its current and future environment: what the body evolved to do and where do we want it to go? Why can't we use our minds to plan and stimulate our bodies to improve how well they perform on a day-to-day basis the functions that they will need for a long healthy life? Why not exploit the fact our bodies respond to our mental input to focus on how to live longer and healthier in an organized way rather than just react to current problems as they arise?

Our advanced mental functions are not being fully utilized if we don't utilize our abilities to forecast future scenarios for our own benefit. We are built to address these issues from an evolutionary perspective where the mindset of the individual is most in sync with our selective evolutionary history that led us here.

Our concepts and ideas, including the metabolism program represented here, do not interfere with any existing fitness modalities but should rather enhance whatever individual sport or fitness endeavors already in place to make the activity more complete. Our health and fitness framework is comprehensive in its scope, taking into account the evolutionary past as well as a lifetime of intentions, plans, choices, and actions. These ideas are based on general scientific principles but refocus them internally to benefit our health and fitness.

Our concepts and programs also embrace all personalized health situations in an individualized way, and programs incorporating IE Fitness are also realistic in their goals and practical in approach. We only seek to give the user the best outcomes within the capacity his or her body is able to provide. With only a shift in mindset and few minutes a day, we can maximize a powerful tool we already use in our minds and focus it toward our own health and fitness.

Visit www.intendedevolution.com to continue your education and find more resources to aid you in your health goals.

The will to live is one of the most powerful instincts we all share; let's use it not to just live, but to live well.

WHO WE ARE

The concepts of Intended Evolution have been used to develop many more visualizations and forms for the important systems of the body, including but not limited to those addressed above. Other systems include cardiovascular, pulmonary, and the central nervous system. We also develop specialized programs for certain demographics or groups, such as wellness programs for office settings or elderly care facilities, diabetes regimes, or even mind-body cancer programs.

While we have not had the opportunity to test our programs scientifically, we have seen remarkable results with our Fit-150 weight-loss and metabolism program, a part of which is described as part of Jane's weight-loss program.

We look forward to the opportunity to partner with an institution or company to study efficacy for metabolism issues and have developed a protocol for a group of patients on diabetic medication. We believe this program would have remarkable results with endpoints that include participants' doctors reducing or eliminating medication.

We hope you have enjoyed and been intrigued by this remarkable new outlook on health and fitness and what it implies. The depth and importance of the mind-body paradigm in all aspects of human physiology has not yet begun to be appreciated. From health, fitness, to our own personal *internal medicine*, each individual has much more control over the future of his or her own health and fitness than most people realize.

These health and fitness concepts and programs were invented by Dr. Don Zhang of Austin, Texas and is based on his theory of Intended Evolution, as put forward in the book of the same name.

The programs invented to date were years in the making and testing, some of which—such as the Fit-150 weight-loss and metabolism program—have been taught recently in Austin, Texas with remarkable anecdotal results for weight loss and diabetes. More ideas will be worked on in the future, and at the present time, the knowledge is being organized and potential research partners or end users being sought by the authors and Live Oak Wellness Concepts, LLC of Austin, Texas.

Live Oak Wellness is considering any number of possibilities for its current and future programs, including licensing, partnering accrediting trainers and fitness experts, and vigorously pursuing outside institutions or groups to run studies on the metabolism program for efficacy in a population of people on diabetic medications. We also believe targeted fat loss, normally thought to be impossible, can be shown with studies on fat remodeling.

We can also help design specially tailored programs and visualizations as adjuncts to existing programs, from muscle building to yoga. However, we strongly believe the metabolism program can prove a very important tool for diabetes and the obesity epidemic in the US today.

Please feel free to contact us about opportunities related to your interests or any questions about what we have presented in the book.

Dr. Dongxun Zhang, DAOM, PhD is the creator of both the theory of intended evolution and the Intended Evolution Fitness System. Zhang is a doctor of acupuncture and oriental medicine (DAOM). He is a professor and member of the doctoral program advisory committee of Texas Health and Science University, is on the faculty of Consilient Innovation Network, and is a former director of the International Association of Integrated Medicine, for whom he has addressed the United Nations. In 1997, he was recognized by the Sixth International Traditional Chinese Medicine Conference with the Hwang Di Award for his microdiagnostic system.

Bob Zhang, LAc was born in China and moved to the United States at the age of ten. He went to middle school, high school, and college in Austin, Texas. He is married and has two children.

David Kincade, LAc holds BS degrees in biology and economics and an MS in Oriental Medicine (MSOM). He practices Oriental Medicine in Austin, Texas.

ENDNOTES

[1] Dongxun Zhang and Bob Zhang. *Intended Evolution.* Austin: River Grove Books, 2015.

[2] Michael Hopkin. "Bacteria 'can learn': Colonies evolve to anticipate changes in their surroundings," *Nature* (May 8, 2008). doi: 10.1038/news.207.360.

[3] "Mind Body Medicine Program." *Georgetown University School of Medicine.* Accessed July 29, 2016. https://som.georgetown.edu/medicaleducation/mindbod.

"Mind-body Medicine." *University of Maryland Medical Center.* Accessed July 29, 2016. http://umm.edu/health/medical/altmed/treatment/mindbody-medicine.

"Mind Body Medicine." *Walter Reed National Military Medical Center.* Accessed July 29, 2016. http://www.wrnmmc.capmed. mil/Health Services/Medicine/Medicine/Internal Medicine/ MindBody/SitePages/Home.aspx.

[4] Barile, Lucio, Isotta Chimenti, Roberto Gaetani, Elvira Forte, Fabio Miraldi, Giacomo Frati, Elisa Messina, and Alessandro Giacomello. "Cardiac Stem Cells: Isolation, Expansion and Experimental Use for Myocardial Regeneration." *Nature Clinical Practice Cardiovascular Medicine* 4 (2007). doi: 10.1038/ncpcardio0738.

Ernst, Aurélie, Kanar Alkass, Samuel Bernard, Mehran Salehpour, Shira Perl, John Tisdale, Göran Possnert, Henrik Druid, and Jonas Frisén. "Neurogenesis in the Striatum of the Adult Human Brain." *Cell* 156, no. 5 (2014): 1072-083. doi: 10.1016/j.cell.2014.01.044.

[5] Dongxun Zhang and Bob Zhang. *Intended Evolution.* Austin: River Grove Books, 2015.

[6] Bely, A. E. "Evolutionary Loss of Animal Regeneration: Pattern and Process." *Integrative and Comparative Biology* 50, no. 4 (2010): 515-27. doi: 10.1093/icb/icq118.

[7] Galera, Andrés. "The Impact of Lamarck's Theory of Evolution Before Darwin's Theory." *Journal of the History of Biology*, 2016. doi: 10.1007/s10739-015-9432-5.

[8] "Where Do We Get Adult Stem Cells?" *Boston Children's Hospital.* Accessed July 29, 2016. http://stemcell.childrenshospital.org/about-stem-cells/adult-somatic-stem-cells-101/where-do-we-get-adult-stem-cells.

[9] McLennan, Deborah A. "The Concept of Co-option: Why Evolution Often Looks Miraculous." *Evolution: Education and Outreach* 1, no. 3 (2008): 247-58. doi: 10.1007/s12052-008-0053-8.

[10] "Coronary Angiogenesis: An Introduction." *Coronary Angiogenesis.* Accessed July 29, 2016. http://biomed.brown.edu/Courses/BI108/BI108_2003_Groups/Coronary_Angiogenesis/BACK.HTM.

[11] Smith, Zachary D., and Alexander Meissner. "DNA Methylation: Roles in Mammalian Development." *Nature Reviews Genetics* 14, no. 3 (2013): 204-20. doi: 10.1038/nrg3354.

[12] Dongxun Zhang and Bob Zhang. *Intended Evolution.* Austin: River Grove Books, 2015.

[13] Schamberger, Andrea C., Claudia A. Staab-Weijnitz, Nikica Mise-Racek, and Oliver Eickelberg. "Cigarette Smoke Alters Primary Human Bronchial Epithelial Cell Differentiation at the Air-liquid Interface." *Scientific Reports* 5 (2015): 8163. doi: 10.1038/srep08163.

[14] Sethi, Prairna. "The Effect of Mindfulness-Based Stress Reduction on Anxiety and Aggression." *New York University Department of Applied Psychology.* Accessed July 29, 2016. http://steinhardt.nyu.edu/appsych/opus/issues/2014/spring/sethi.

Chiesa, Alberto, and Alessandro Serretti. "Mindfulness-Based Stress Reduction for Stress Management in Healthy People: A Review and Meta-Analysis." *The Journal of Alternative and Complementary Medicine* 15, no. 5 (2009): 593-600. doi: 10.1089/acm.2008.0495.

[15] "Mind-body Medicine." *University of Maryland Medical Center.* Accessed July 29, 2016. http://umm.edu/health/medical/altmed/treatment/mindbody-medicine.

[16] Larkin, Kevin T. *Stress and Hypertension: Examining the Relation between Psychological Stress and High Blood Pressure.* New Haven: Yale University Press, 2005.

[17] Randall, Michael. "The Physiology of Stress: Cortisol and the Hypothalamic-Pituitary-Adrenal Axis." *Dartmouth Undergraduate Journal of Science Online.* February 03, 2011. Accessed July 29, 2016. http://dujs.dartmouth.edu/2011/02/the-physiology-of-stress-cortisol-and-the-hypothalamic-pituitary-adrenal-axis/#.V4gN-ldgpFI.

"Hormones: Communication between the Brain and the Body." *Brain Facts.* April 1, 2012. Accessed July 29, 2016. http://www.brainfacts.org/brain-basics/cell-communication/articles/2012/hormones-communication-between-the-brain-and-the-body.

[18] Zadra, Jonathan R., and Gerald L. Clore. "Emotion and Perception: The Role of Affective Information." *Wiley Interdisciplinary Reviews: Cognitive Science* 2, no. 6 (2011): 676-85. doi: 10.1002/wcs.147.

[19] Bray, Molly S. "Implications of Gene-Behavior Interactions: Prevention and Intervention for Obesity." *Obesity* 16 (2008). doi: 10.1038/oby.2008.522.

[20] "Obesity Linked with Mood and Anxiety Disorders." *NIMH RSS.* July 3, 2006. Accessed July 29, 2016. http://www.nimh.nih.gov/news/science-news/2006/obesity-linked-with-mood-and-anxiety-disorders.shtml.

21 Price, Michael. "The Risks of Night Work." *American Psychological Association*. January 2011. Accessed July 29, 2016. http://www.apa.org/monitor/2011/01/night-work.aspx.

22 Gilbert, Scott F. *Ecological Developmental Biology: The Environmental Regulation of Development, Health, and Evolution.* Sunderland, MA: Sinauer Associates, 2015.

23 O'Keefe, James H., Harshal R. Patil, Carl J. Lavie, Anthony Magalski, Robert A. Vogel, and Peter A. Mccullough. "Potential Adverse Cardiovascular Effects from Excessive Endurance Exercise." *Mayo Clinic Proceedings* 87, no. 6 (2012): 587-95. doi: 10.1016/j.mayocp.2012.04.005.

24 Dongxun Zhang and Bob Zhang. "The Life Cycle: Why Do We Die?" *Intended Evolution.* Austin: River Grove Books, 2015.

25 Windsor, Tim D., Rachel G. Curtis, and Mary A. Luszcz. "Sense of Purpose as a Psychological Resource for Aging Well." *Developmental Psychology* 51, no. 7 (2015): 975-86. doi: 10.1037/dev0000023.
"Working Longer May Lead to a Longer Life, New OSU Research Shows." *Oregon State University.* Accessed July 29, 2016. <http://oregonstate.edu/ua/ncs/archives/2016/apr/working-longer-may-lead-longer-life-new-osu-research-shows>.

26 Phillips, David P., Camilla A. Van Voorhees, and Todd E. Ruth. "The Birthday: Lifeline or Deadline?" *Psychosomatic Medicine* 54, no. 5 (1992): 532–542. doi: 10.1097/00006842-199209000-00001.

27 "Albert Brown (American Veteran)." *Wikipedia.* Accessed October 11, 2016. https://en.wikipedia.org/wiki/Albert_Brown_(American_veteran).

[28] Sedwick, Caitlin. "Yoshinori Ohsumi: Autophagy from Beginning to End." *Journal of Cell Biology*. April 16, 2012. Accessed October 11, 2016. http://jcb.rupress.org/content/197/2/164.

[29] Gilbert, Scott F. *Ecological Developmental Biology: The Environmental Regulation of Development, Health, and Evolution*. Sunderland, MA: Sinauer Associates, 2015.

[30] Williams, D., A. Kuipers, C. Mukai, and R. Thirsk. "Acclimation during Space Flight: Effects on Human Physiology." *Canadian Medical Association Journal* 180, no. 13 (2009): 1317-323. doi: 10.1503/cmaj.090628.

[31] Telles, Shirley, Patricia Gerbarg, and Elisa H. Kozasa. "Physiological Effects of Mind and Body Practices." *BioMed Research International* 2015 (2015): 1-2. doi: 10.1155/2015/983086.

[32] Spino, Michael P., and William F. Straub. "Effect of Mental Training on the Performance of College Age Distance Runners." *The Sport Journal*. Accessed July 29, 2016. http://thesportjournal.org/article/effect-of-mental-training-on-the-performance-of-college-age-distance-runners.

[33] Spino, Michael P., and William F. Straub. "Effect of Mental Training on the Performance of College Age Distance Runners." *The Sport Journal*. Accessed July 29, 2016. http://thesportjournal.org/article/effect-of-mental-training-on-the-performance-of-college-age-distance-runners.

Parnabas, Vincent, Julinamary Parnabas, and Antoinette Mary Parnabas. "Internal and External Imagery on Sports Performance among Swimmers." *European Academic Research* 2, no. 11 (2015): 14735–14741.

[34] Spino, Michael P., and William F. Straub. "Effect of Mental Training on the Performance of College Age Distance Runners." *The Sport Journal.* Accessed July 29, 2016. http://thesportjournal.org/article/effect-of-mental-training-on-the-performance-of-college-age-distance-runners.

[35] Klein, Stanley B., and Shaun Nichols. "Memory and the Sense of Personal Identity." *Mind* 121, no. 483 (2012): 677-702. doi: 10.1093/mind/fzs080.

[36] Stahl, James E., Michelle L. Dossett, A. Scott Lajoie, John W. Denninger, Darshan H. Mehta, Roberta Goldman, Gregory L. Fricchione, and Herbert Benson. "Relaxation Response and Resiliency Training and Its Effect on Healthcare Resource Utilization." *PLOS ONE* 10, no. 10 (2015). doi: 10.1371/journal.pone.0140212.

[37] Dewar, Gwen. "The Cognitive Benefits of Play: Effects on the Learning Brain." *Parenting Science.* Accessed July 29, 2016. http://www.parentingscience.com/benefits-of-play.html.

White, Rachel E. "The Power of Play: A Research Summary on Play and Learning." *Minnesota Children's Museum.* Fall 2012. Accessed July 29, 2016. http://www.childrensmuseums.org/images/MCMResearchSummary.pdf.

[38] Dongxun Zhang and Bob Zhang. "The Information Cycle." *Intended Evolution.* Austin: River Grove Books, 2015.

[39] Coelho, Marisa, Teresa Oliveira, and Ruben Fernandes. "Biochemistry of Adipose Tissue: An Endocrine Organ." *Archives of Medical Science* 2 (2013): 191-200. doi: 10.5114/aoms.2013.33181.

Made in the USA
San Bernardino, CA
24 May 2017